Still Living
the Best Life
I Ever Had

Gerry Williamson

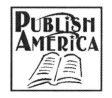

PublishAmerica
Baltimore

First printing

ISBN: 1-4241-6444-3
PUBLISHED BY PUBLISHAMERICA, LLLP
www.publishamerica.com
Baltimore

Printed in the United States of America

To those living with traumatic brain injury—
only they know what it's like.

I thank God for keeping I me alive to write this.
I thank Taylor for saying I should write a book about my life.
I thank Edith Bowman for writing the foreword
and all the editing she did.
I thank Marty for doing lots of editing.
I thank Shirley McKenzie for the finest of details.
I thank Aunty Wava for the finest of details.
I thank Gordon Watts for giving me my first computer because using
a computer helps people with traumatic brain injury.
I thank Redge for the computer help he gave me.
I thank Cheryl Asbia for the computer help she gave me.
I thank David West for some editing.
I thank Hella and PublishAmerica for being there

Preface

Gerry Williamson. This man. This paradox. This remarkable, unremarkable man. This extraordinary, ordinary man—born into a humble enough beginning, thrown young into heartbreak, agony, disaster, tremendous personal loss, disability and nightmare, faced with odds of unbearable proportion. This is his tale, told with humility but with glory, of, most importantly of all, his long battle too against the legacy of traumatic brain injury, well fought and deservedly won, but with its remnants and other arenas awaiting its continuation.

This fighter. This survivor. This inspiration to thousands upon thousands of other ordinary men and women facing similar challenges now presents his story as between friends, in his own inimitable and unique style of writing—chatting to a beloved personal friend—the reader.

I have known Gerry for but a relatively few years, but in that time have learned of his indomitable spirit, his determination and, above all, his compassion—his desire to learn, and success in learning from his own experiences, not with self-pity or anger, but as a gift of understanding of others and of giving them an infection of hope for a future thought lost and restored. This is a human of superhuman humanity. When he asked me to provide a preface for his story, for his offering of his most intimate thoughts, experiences and message, I accepted without hesitation, realising fully the privilege he was offering to me, and the honour he was granting.

Read this tale with belief in that message. Read it with an open mind and with willingness to receive inspiration and reassurance of your own ability and strength to meet whatever happens head-on and with the determination to succeed in beating the odds. And, like him, to never give up on your existence and yourself.

I have heard it said that we are all, each one of us, unique. And that no-one should be classed as disabled, but as merely less able. To my mind, Gerry is amongst the most unique and is far more able than I in so many ways. We are thousands of miles apart in geographical terms, me in the Old World, he in the New. But one promise I can make is that by the time you have finished reading his story, you will be good neighbours, the miles between having been dissolved by nothing more than identification with circumstances and experiences.

So read, and enjoy. Take time to get into his mind and heart, and take courage and strength from what you read. Gerry—thank you for allowing the world to share these few thousand words with you.

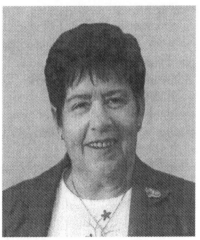

Edith O. Bowman FRICS, ILTM

Lecturer in Law and Estate Management
School of the Built Environment
Heriot—Wat University
Edinburgh, Scotland, UK

Foreword

In what you're about to read, I have stayed as close to the truth as I possibly can because I know I won't have to remember what I've said if I always tell the truth.

Like most live-wires (those people who are always looking for something to do) I too was far too busy living my life the wrong way to write down what I was doing in it to give an accurate accounting of my life until I was into my fifth decade. That was when I thought loudly to myself: "That sure was quick." It's also when I asked myself, "What happened?"

Life didn't go the way I thought it would. At least it didn't go the way I thought it should.

I know that people want to make their own mistakes themselves because they think they are different than everybody else.

I thought I was different too.

Today I see I'm an expert on myself and I don't have to pretend I'm someone else anymore. I've convinced myself a shade past a shadow of doubt that when things seemed too good to be true they usually were. From that I realized what was in life in the beginning stays to the end, and because I didn't come into this world with any weapons, I'd have to teach myself to use my brain to defend myself.

I also wrote this book because I'd like my life to be counted as something important in the scheme of things, and refreshing memories in other people's minds is a feast for sure. Seeing how I'm like you there might be a few things you thought were closer to fiction than fact. And as you know, fact is sometimes stranger than fiction. They'll have to do when I've turned to dust.

Sometimes, when the most important things were happening, I wasn't paying attention to what was going on. So I've had to rely on what other people said happened, and what they've told me splashed onto other ideas that caused different memories to flow into streams of thought that made me think these facts were the highest highs, the lowest lows and the biggest big deals of my life.

If you've already found you've followed the wrong path in your own life, and think it's impossible to cross the mountains of doubt you're now faced with, you might find they were only foothills when you've digested some of the peaks I've crossed. More people have died climbing molehills, thinking they were mountains, than I've got fingers and toes to count them with.

Something I discovered when I tried to remember things from the past were those memories grabbed hold of other thoughts, turning themselves into rabbits that kept running and running to keep my dream of becoming a writer alive.

I feel that I've been kept alive for a reason, maybe for you to read what I've written. Lots of people have seen how my life has gone, but this is how I feel it went.

Some dates may be a little off, but that's only proof I'm human. And in discovering that I've also discovered the way I was intended to be.

Gerry Williamson

My First Life

Chapter 1
His Belly Button

Flying Phil, was a young, stud-faced 'hogger' (nickname, or as I like to think of that word, 'nicker') working as a railway engineer on the Canadian Pacific Railway in the 1940s. He earned that sarcastic nicker of his by running his locomotive slowly because he knew an engine's power was stronger than the ability to stop a sneeze. If an automobile was ever on the tracks and he knew he couldn't steer around it—the locomotive always won.

Whenever this happened, as it occasionally did, it became the biggest regret Phil had about his job. Though he was a careful engineer, Phil must have been a lousy drinker when he was younger because I was such a lousy drinker when I was that age. That's probably why he rarely drank when he was older—the memories of the past were still sticking to his thoughts.

Phil was holding his 'stuff' together while rooming and boarding at a house for single men in Revelstoke, British Columbia. Instead of going out drinking and carousing with the other railway workers all the time, he preferred going out for a cup of coffee instead. When he was working afternoons and his 'quit' was good enough (a quit is getting off work early because all his work was finished early) he'd hustle his way to the only cafe still open that late at night.

There was a spunky young waitress working at that restaurant whose birth name was misspelled into Margarrette because her dad didn't know how to spell that well. But she had been nickered Adie in her youth by her neighbourhood friends because she had a nun named Sister Mary-Adrian for an aunt. When she had grown out of her youth she found herself working as a waitress in the same restaurant Phil frequented. One night, when it was dark and spooky out, Phil asked if he could walk her to her boarding house as a gentlemanly gesture. This impressed Adie to forever.

In conversation along the way they discovered they had more in common than smoking the same brand of plain-end cigarettes and soon fell in love.

As the slow drool of time moved them into the future, they traveled to St. Pat's (St. Patrick's Church) in Vancouver to hear wedding bells announcing they were now man and wife. After honeymooning around Vancouver for a week or so, and returned to Revelstoke, they started living in a larger room in a boarding house.

Mom and Dad are the couple on left in their wedding picture.

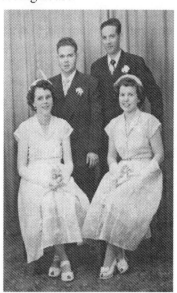

Time passed, and my sister, Jackie, was born and a few years later my life began in Revelstoke's Queen Victoria Hospital on my Aunty Wava's thirty-first birthday on July 10, 1952.

From the beginning, my thinking told me I was starving to death, so a lady with milk-swollen breasts (whose baby had died) offered me hers for nourishment, causing my internal instincts to drool over what any other breast-sucking baby wants to do with an offered bosom. Mom didn't know that woman had a future blood-donating-destroying case of Hepatitis-A inside her—making it impossible for me to give blood to this day.

When time had passed and I was issued my first set of memories, Mom casually mentioned that the night before my birth she overheard a drunken Flying Phil telling his friend, 'If Adie has a son, I'm going to name him after you!' Giving me the distinction of being named after a drunken Gerry.

Dad was forced to move to Notchhill, BC, for a few months and then he had to move to the only other place in BC where he had enough seniority to hold a job, Vancouver. He stayed with my grandparents (Mom and Pop Steeple, who had adopted Phil from an orphanage and moved to what was going to be the capital of BC at one time—Fort Langly) until arrangements could be made to move the other three members of my family to a rented house on Rindall Avenue on the south side of what CP Rail called Westminster Junction, but thought of as Port Coquitlam by the people living there.

I was stuck on automatic pilot for my first few years of life because I was so stunned to be alive. Today, I'm still not sure if it was that first two-year-old's mouthful of stolen beer I'd drank from an unwatched bottle or what it was that made me think the way I would always think—all I know is that I spent my first few summers of my life tied to the clothesline in the backyard so I could run some excess energy off in an attempt to control me better.

For every bad thing that happens in life there is always something good that balances it out. The good thing that happened in my life at that time was a brother named Terry born on April 13, 1954, at the Royal Columbian Hospital in New Westminster. With Terry's inclusion in the family there were now three of us kids playing in the branches of our family tree—bringing the total number of mouths to feed up to five. I got jealous of all the care and attention being fluffed on him because I missed the concentration of attention that used to be powdered on me and did whatever made Mom or Dad pay more attention to me.

When I was around three years old I put a garbage can over my head when playing on the swings in the backyard, and because I wasn't holding on when I should have been, I fell off with a scream. Mom flew out the back door when she heard all the commotion I was making, and found me lying on the ground with the garbage can still over my head screaming like an ambulance. She started to take the can off my head but I wouldn't let her because I was afraid my head would come off with it. So she was forced to carry Terry on her hip with Jackie leading me by the hand along the wooden sidewalk that covered the potholes that were on the southern end of Shaughnessy Street to the doctor's office with the garbage can still over my head.

Another attention-grabbing time, after Mom and Dad had done their grocery shopping for the coming week, I got out of bed before everyone else did and peeled off every label of every can in the pantry for something to do. This turned meal times into an unwanted adventure for Mom because it forced her to try and guess the contents of every can before she opened them.

In the Rindall Avenue house the stairs to the second floor were a few paces away from the front door against the wall. The wallpaper on the wall at the foot of the steps was peeling, and one day I decided to trim that curling paper by burning the loose ends off. Because I was older than Terry he always watched everything I did because he wanted to know what to do when presented with the same things. Big brother worship was in there too. All of a sudden, the rest of the paper on the wall felt sympathy for the burning paper and danced into flame as well. Seeing this and knowing Terry couldn't move as fast as I could, I ran away yelling that Terry had set the wall on fire. He got his fingers burnt for that, and because he didn't fink (or rat me out) when he knew who had set the fire, I never got caught. Having said that: I've just been released from feeling guilty about something that happened a long time ago by telling you the truth, or as I like think of it, by 'truthing you.'

One day I walked a block from our house to a chicken coop that was behind a house beside a dairy on Pitt River Road, to watch the owners feeding the chickens. But I got there too late and was left feeling sorry for myself looking at the chickens moving around the pen searching for food. All of a sudden a great big mouse caught my eye. I'd never seen such a big mouse before, and when it realized I'd seen it, it stopped moving. So I dropped a rock on it to get it to move again. I was so sure I rocked it dead that I stuck my hand inside the pen and picked it up. But that mouse turned into a rat playing possum, and bit me on the knuckle of my right thumb where a scar remains to remind me of what happened. Seeing all that blood and feeling all that pain made me run for home as fast as I could—hooting and hollering that a great big mouse had bit me. Successfully ending my first time out of the yard on my own on a sour note. This started my long jagged career of stepping on rusty nails and getting tetanus shots.

Dad decided Mom was walking to the doctor's office too much and convinced himself that she should learn how to drive the family car. She got her learners-license and Dad along with Mom's best friend, Shirley, taught her how to drive. Because family unity would be dissolved if the rest of the family stayed at home, we kids went along for the ride. I still remember the amount of fear playing behind my belly button—I'll be referring to as 'scaredy-cats' for the rest of your read here—when I was sitting in the back seat of the car as Mom took over the driving duties. I was so scared that I had to get out of the car and go number one against a tree. As an added bonus to this self-inflicted scaredy cat I managed to slam the car door solidly on my own fingers when getting back in the car, and blubbered about it all the way home, adding to the short but growing list of trauma in my life.

Another agitation that entered my life at this time started when another boy, named Allan, saw something he didn't like about himself reflected off of me, and made it a point to punch me in the nose or kick me in the prick every time he saw me in typical bully fashion. This happened so much over the years that the damage to my nose was never repaired; guaranteeing the septum in my left nostril remained deviated to this day.

In the 1950s everything was cheaper than it is today, and to try and shave some of the hyper-activeness off me Dad bought a little hammer and a bucket of nails for me to beat into a stump sticking out of the ground in the backyard. Dad wanted my nailing to look as neat as this:

```
        .
       . .
      . . .
    . . . . .
  . . . . . . .
```

But I gave up trying for neatness and hammered the nails in any way they wanted to go in and my nailing came out looking like this:

```
        ?
      . V ./
     .\ / . / .\
     / . . . \ .
   . \ . \ . / . . instead.
```

When the Shell gas station started operation on the corner of Shaughnessy and Pitt River Road, Shell Oil sent everyone in that area a key to try and open a lock that was on a safe at the station as an incentive to use Shell gas. The station was only a block away from our house and two or three times a day I'd go there and try all the keys that were thrown away after other people had tried them. One day I opened the lock and an alarm went off. I was positive I had broken it and I grabbed the key and ran home. Later that same day when Mom and Dad tried their key and the same thing happened, our family won a Coleman Stove and I won my first tricycle, which the owner of the gas station, Mister C, wasn't going to let me have at first.

A foster brother nickered 'Go' started living with us about now, raising the number of family members to six. Terry's life began as normally as any other little boy's started. But as time closed the door on his babyhood and opened the gate to his boyhood, a few negative characteristics started showing themselves off in his make-up kit—as I like to think of the way he was. He had difficulty going up and down stairs, and he had a slight waddle when he walked being the most obvious.

Around this time my bad temper over not getting my own way made me hit another kid over the head with my hammer, giving him a scar that will last as long as his belly button.

Chapter 2
Lucifer

In August 1958, I started getting upset about starting to go to Central Elementary School in September. That was the first time I realized I was getting older and it was the first time I started worrying about it.

My first teacher, Miss Neufeld, was patient with me when I was having such a hard time adjusting to my life as a new student. She told us little kids about our part of the school by saying, "This little room is called the cloak-room, where you hang your coats up on these little pegs and put your lunches in the boxes above them when you first come to school in the morning." She explained everything to us the way you would explain things to a five- or six-year-old; that now that we were starting school we'd have to raise our hands and ask permission if we wanted to go to the bathroom. When she said that I wondered if we were supposed to start doing that at home too.

She went into great detail telling us about how the fire bells worked and what happened when they rang. All it took was hearing that fire trucks would start racing to the school with their sirens screaming for everyone to 'GET OUT OF THE WAY' and volunteer firemen (as I thought firefighters were called in those days) hanging onto the back of the trucks for dear life (as they did in those days too) for my mind to start thinking of all the possibilities that could happen with that bit of information. Right then and there plans started lining up behind each other to pull the alarm.

I'd never been with as many kids my own age before and i of being like everyone else I made myself different than ther because I thought I was different than everyone—I was differer knew that I had to learn how to operate that fire alarm by mys I would never know how it worked.

My mind convinced me I had to go to the bathroom so I put my up and walked out of the class the way I was told to do. But i explained that I was supposed to ask permission before I left the i After the alarm started singing it sang so loudly that it shocked m scratching my head and fluttering my lips in confusion. I w surprised at how loud it rang that I was left standing there with the of it streaming from my eyes—letting my tears tell everybody l responsible for the volunteer firemen leaving their jobs to gallop t school in such a hurry. It was more than obvious who made the a sing like it was doing because of all the broken glass around my The principal of the school, Mr. D., told the firemen what happe and the trucks left. I was so upset that they didn't leave with t sirens wailing like they were doing when they arrived that I sta crying.

When we were back in the classroom, it was explained what were going to be doing for the rest of the year. I was now a good li boy—contenting myself with looking out the window at all the c flowing by the school in single file and listening to the questions be asked by the other kids in the classroom. I was looking out the wind and because I didn't see any fire trucks going by, I put my hand uf go to the bathroom. I was warned not to pull the alarm again and w out into the hallway. I made it all the way into the room I'd been tc only boys could go into, and paused in thought over why everybo used the same bathroom at home but used separate ones at scho

I was looking at how big the bathroom was when I saw the uri n for the first time. I didn't know how to work it and used the toi l instead, and walked back into the hallway. When I got out there a attention-getting bird-brained idea chirped into my ear to pull the ala r again. So I did.

All my classmates came out into the hallway with Miss Neufeld pulling up the rear. As she walked by me she asked, "Did you do that?" I nodded yes, and she went to tell Mr. D. that it was another false alarm. As a reward for doing what I'd done, I was taken to his office and given a licking across the bum, stamping my first day of school as the first time I got the strap there.

A few months later after bumping my head against the wall where my desk was, and feeling it didn't hurt and finding the sound it made inside my head fascinated me so much I bumped it again and again—holding my jaw tight and loose listening to the different sounds inside my head. I did this for a few minutes before Miss Neufeld asked me what I thought I was doing. I didn't know what else to say, so I truthed her by saying, "I like hearing the sound it makes inside my head when I do that," turning me into an extrovert.

That was the first time I heard people laugh at something I said at school. I couldn't understand what was so funny but I loved the attention it gave me. It made me happy to know that I could make everybody laugh like that, that I started thinking that school wasn't that bad after all and the class clown in me was born—because I discovered I had a captive audience.

When I took my first report card home, this is what Mom and Dad read: "Gerry's progress is hampered by his poor attitude. He has made discoveries that he can succeed if he tries, but he has not overcome his poor attitude as of yet."

I settled down after getting that comment by getting perfect attendance for my second report card. But in the third I missed a week because I had to have my tonsils and adenoids taken out because they were infected. Go said I had to get them out because I probably drank out of the toilet too much.

The rest of the marks on that report card were mainly N's for normal, with the odd U, for unsatisfactory, tossed into the cauldron of subjects like spelling, reading, arithmetic and printing (which is still bad.) The general behaviour and work habit parts on most of my elementary report cards were hammered down with hardy U's, demonstrating that I was full of sensitivity even at that young age.

Throughout the rest of that school year I did a lot of things that were not thought of as bad bad by the teacher, but were considered bad in the unruly, not well-behaved department of doing things. I was always doing things that bugged the teacher: squirming around in my seat, and talking out of turn, etc. In other words I was a pain in the back pocket. Somehow I passed that first year of school by the skin of my teeth, and in the summer of 1959 our family moved across the railway tracks to the north side of town and started living in a rented house on Salisbury Avenue. This house didn't have a barn taking up most of the backyard, but half was taken up by lawn, and the other half was left uncluttered by neatness for Dad to plant a garden.

Whenever Terry walked anywhere he would trip over things that weren't there. This slowed the family down whenever we walked anywhere. As he was getting older, he tried running like the other kids in the neighbourhood, but he ran so bowlegged that he'd fall down because his running looked more awkward than his walking.

Sometime during the summer between grades one and two I started squinting and Mom or Dad noticed what I was doing and took me to see an eye doctor. This doctor said my eyes were fine but were lazy, meaning I turned my head rather than my eyes when I wanted to see something. I was given some eye exercises to do every day to make them stronger, and I started wearing glasses with corrective lenses in them to force my eyes to look at things in a different way. I did those eye exercises every day for two months before I quit doing them because no one was making sure I was. The marks I was getting on those report-cards caused my grade-two teacher to get so concerned about me that she warned Mom and Dad that I'd better improve my marks or I'd have to repeat the entire school year. I thought they were only kidding about getting better marks and didn't try to improve anything. After repeatedly being warned I'd have to do grade two again, and repeatedly ignoring the requests to improve my marks, I was told I had to do the year over again. My reward for flunking that year was to be sent to summer school, that I went to every summer until I was finished with the fourth grade. Making number two my lucky number. I didn't like going to summer school because some of the other kids going there with me seemed to be slower thinkers than me and couldn't understand what I understood.

Terry started going to school in September 1960, and Jackie, Terry and I would leave the house at the same time every morning. This ailment of Terry's made him stop walking every so often to wait for some fresh energy to build up inside him to give him the strength to make it the rest of the way to Viscount. He was constantly stopping and talking to perfectly good strangers along the way and because this slowed Jackie and me down and because I was so impatient, I'd scoot ahead of them. The dormant 'mother's instinct' in Jackie's personality started showing itself off this year by making sure that Terry made it to his classroom okay.

Seeing Terry's lack of coordination increasing and realizing he couldn't do things the way their other two kids did them upset Mom and Dad; it confused them so much that it started dominating their thoughts and overflowed into their conversations with friends. Mom and Shirley would often talk about Terry's demeanour. In fact, it was Shirley who determined the name of what Terry's problem was years before the family doctor did.

This fully trained and highly paid doctor that examined Terry told Mom that lots of kids go through stages like that, and usually outgrew this physical drawback in a few years. This doctor also said that Mom and Dad were probably babying him too much because he was the youngest of the family. These theories served up a birdhouse full of woodpeckers that pecked at Mom and Dad's thoughts for the next few years because that answer they were given acted like a placebo in their thoughts by making them feel better without doing anything about the problem.

In September 1960, when my second year in grade two began, I thought I was smarter than everyone else in the class because I'd already been through grade two once already. I didn't think I'd failed because I wasn't smart enough, but flunked because I couldn't communicate with the tests we were being given. I've always felt that, but didn't know how to communicate it to myself until I got older and could nimble my way around words easier. This was the third flock of kids I'd flown with and I felt a little nervous that they were younger than me that I spent a lot of time looking out the classroom window until Mom and Dad saw the first report card I got that year. A request from the teacher to see my parents was answered by a visit from the disciplinarian of the household. And when Mom went to that meeting she was told everything I'd been doing in class. When she came home after it, she bawled me out so much that I was forced to smarten up. By the time 1961 was a reality, I was getting straight N's in all my classes.

Mom had been a leader, called Baloo (the Bear) in the 1st Port Coquitlam Cub pack on the south side of town for a few years and had asked me to join her group. Cub leaders were named after characters in *The Jungle Book* by the way. I went with her a few times, but didn't want to keep going because the cub pack met on the other side of town and I didn't have any friends living on that side of town anymore.

Every 'May Day' (Port Coquitlam's annual fair) when it was being held in 'Aggie Park'—nickered that because there was a community hall called the Agricultural Hall there at one time—where you can find the Kinsmen Centre today, across the street from where the wading pool was, that is being used for a planter in McMitchell Park today—close to where the Cenotaph originally was. At this fair I'd always bump into Allan and his friends, guys that were too afraid of him not to be his friend, and every time I saw him I'd freeze because I hoped he didn't see me. But he invariably did, and I'd always leave the park with a bloody nose or sore privates.

My Uncle Buck was my godfather who worked as a lineman. He used thick leather belts to climb wooden telephone poles to repair the electric wires and could afford to buy what he called 'elephant's milk' for his family to drink, which turned out to be homogenized milk. Our family drank powdered milk that we made our selves and always tasted watered down. One day Uncle Buck gave Mom and Dad part of a thick leather belt that he wasn't using for climbing telephone poles anymore because it was starting to crack. The reason he gave it to them was so they could use it on my bum or hands, since Mom and Dad were always telling him about the escapades I was pulling off. I don't know who came up with the nicker for the belt, and it really doesn't matter today, because I still get a slight shiver running up my spine whenever my thoughts snag a glimpse of 'Lucifer.'

Chapter 3
Catastrophe

When I went back to Viscount in September 1962 I felt like a big shot in my grade-four class because my birthday had been in the summer and my age was now double digits. I was ten. I got my first man teacher that year, and it seemed like Mr. B. took great pride in smacking some of us grade-fours on the hands when we were bad. I'm not sure if I should be proud or embarrassed by this, but I got whacked on the hands the first day of school for something I'd done. Ironically I never got whipped (got the strap from the principal) all year because Mr. B. liked to take care of broken rules right in his classroom.

As far as I was concerned the most important thing that I learned this year was my ability to look out the classroom window while listening to what was being talked about in the class.

I became aware of television this year, but I still wasn't all that excited about it, because TV wasn't that good at that time and I only watched it because it was there, or the occasional good program was on it. We never had to worry about what program we'd watch because the only channels we could get at that time were channels 2, 6 and 12. And most of the time it looked like it was snowing on what we were watching but we'd watch it like that anyway.

If it was ever windy outside and we were having bad reception on the TV Go would usually go outside and turn the TV aerial that was attached to a long pole on the side of the house to get the picture back into focus, while someone else stood by the front door and relayed how the reception was changing according to the viewer in the rumpus room. Seeing how Terry couldn't do stairs that well, I'd usually have to stand at the top of the stairs to pass the messages of how the reception was improving to Go.

Every year one of my favourite movies, *The Wizard of Oz*, was shown on TV and every year we'd gather around our black-and-white TV and watch that great movie. The best part of the show was watching the witch melting.

Now that I was ten I was old enough to walk the block to the corner store by myself whenever Mom or Dad wanted something. I never refused to go when they asked me to because I gave myself the false impression that I was being told to go when I was actually being asked to go. They would usually ask me to get a pack of smokes for them, and I'd always ask if I could keep the change. If they said I could, I'd happily walk up the back alley and go to the Prairie Market. When they said I couldn't, I'd take my time going there or I'd walk the two or three extra blocks and go to the KY Market that was near the corner of Flint and Prairie at that time. This was the year I started to be friendly with corner-store owners as well.

Along with being old enough to go to the store by myself came the added responsibility of having to do chores every day. My main chore was burning the papers in the old oil drum in the backyard, and emptying the wet garbage into the garbage cans beside it. One time I found an old paint can and stuck a stick in the hole in the lid and held it over the open flames—the way you'd do a wiener in a weenie-roast—to see what would happen.

When all of a sudden whooooooooooooooooooooooooooosh! I went in the house with singed eyebrows and hair.

Dad got me to join his Cub pack in 1962, because he was Kaa (the snake) in it, which met in the gym at Viscount every Tuesday night. Cubs got me out of the house at least one night out of the week. Mom and Dad probably hoped it would stop my constant acting up in other situations. Another way of curbing my behavior of constantly fooling around was done by sending us kids to church every Sunday morning for a couple of hours while Mom and Dad stayed at home and did chores around the house. We'd go to the Sunday school part of the services on the ground floor first in order to learn Bible stories and then we'd go upstairs and join the rest of the congregation. We were given thirty-five cents each to put into the collection basket before we left the house. On the weeks I didn't get my allowance because I'd misbehaved too much, I'd sometimes have a little money left in my pocket after putting a quarter in the basket.

Everybody but one person on the south side of town had forgotten all about me, and Allan continued to clobber me every time he saw me. This happened so often over the next few years that I stopped telling Mom and Dad about it because they couldn't do anything about it anyway and I moved into a state of perpetual scaredy-cats whenever I was in public until I was a teenager.

When I got to school in the morning there always seemed to be a bunch of guys around my age playing some game on the big playing field behind Viscount. I was lousy at sports in physical education, but decided I wanted to play soccer or football at the start of the school year and baseball near the end of the school year and started hanging around these guys in the hopes that I'd be asked to play because I realized I'd always wanted to play a physical game with someone at home, and never had anyone in my family to play them with. One day I was asked if I wanted to play football with these guys because they were short a couple of players since it was during Port Coquitlam's unofficial Rain Festival (which runs from October 1 to September 30 every year). Because I'd convinced myself not to let the fact that it was raining control what I really wanted to do, I decided I wanted to play sports outside.

Every morning, recess and lunch hour, rain, snow or shine after that, I'd be out on that big grass field behind Viscount playing whatever sport the guy who got the ball liked best. If they liked soccer better, we'd get a soccer ball. If they liked football best, we got a football, and we'd play 'touch football' until the warning bell rang. When I first started playing sports I'd usually be one of the last people picked to join a team because I was such a lousy player. Gradually, I became one of the first picked.

Jackie always seemed to be too busy upstairs helping the school librarian at lunchtime to know or care to know what I was up to on the playing fields. This didn't matter to me because I was enjoying myself playing sports. I liked sports so much during the week that I started playing soccer on an organized team that played on that same field on the weekends. I enjoyed playing soccer on the weekend so much because I could get out of the house earlier in the morning without having to do chores around the house all day long. I had spent enough time sitting on the players' bench on these organized teams to know I had to be a good player every time I played or I wouldn't be asked to play the next time. I put playing goal at the top of my preference list because a goalie didn't have to run around as much as everyone else did. Besides, it seemed that no one else wanted to play that position because they thought playing goal was boring. I liked playing that position because it would almost guarantee I'd get to play nearly every game.

Jackie finished going to elementary school and started going to PoCo (nicker for Port Coquitlam Junior Senior Secondary School) in September 1962.

Whenever Terry made up his mind he wanted to do anything he'd try his hardest to do it. Like the time he wanted to ride a bicycle; he'd been borrowing other people's bicycles every chance he could get for a few years because he wanted to see for himself if it was even possible to ride a bike. The people who saw him walking thought it would be impossible for him to ride a bicycle because his walking looked so unsteady. But once he got going on one he stopped looking like a sailor before they got their land legs and proved how wrong everybody was by riding surprisingly well. It gave him the freedom to do what he wanted to do when he wanted to do it. Mom and Dad were so impressed by his ability to ride a bike better than he could walk that they bought him a little red one of his own. It immediately became his best friend because he was always riding it wherever there were no hills to go up because hills were too hard on him.

That winter Terry was having a harder time walking to school than usual because of all the snow on the ground. His teacher reacted to his lateness by sending a note home with him suggesting he leave the house earlier to get to school on time. He started leaving the house five minutes before Jackie and I left but we would usually find him sitting on the ground and talking to people, having a short rest, and he had to leave the house ten minutes before we did.

In late May of 1963 I started playing baseball on one of the organized teams that met on the baseball diamonds behind Viscount. I preferred playing soccer because the soccer coach always gave us slices of oranges at half-time, and all the baseball coach let us have were lungs full of fresh air.

Every springtime, my head would get plugged up with snot, and my eyes became itchy, and I was constantly sneezing when mowing the grass in the yard, especially the backyard because it was so big. I'd come in the house with my eyes running like faucets and barely being able to catch my breath for a few minutes. Mom and Dad became concerned about this and mentioned it to the family doctor, who referred me to a specialist in New Westminster because it was suspected I had hay fever or asthma.

This specialist put little scratches on the insides of my arms, and then he put little drops of everything I might be allergic to on these abrasions. The scratches that showed a reaction determined the allergies I had. It was decided I'd start getting booster shots (injections) in the arm) at Leigh Square Medical Centre—the medical centre that our family went to—every Monday, Wednesday and Friday for the next five years when I would start taking less shots until I grew out of these allergies. Getting those shots stopped me from having to mow the grass all the time; it also made everyone in my family think I had to stop playing on grass because of my condition. I wanted to believe them, so I quit playing sports. But after walking on grass a few times I found I wasn't bothered as much as everyone was saying I would be getting because I found that whenever I did walk on grass my head wasn't getting plugged up like I was being told it would be getting and figured I only had to sprint short distances on grass when I was playing goal and wouldn't have to run around that much.

The 1963-64 school year found me upstairs in Mrs. Horne's grade-five classroom. I thought the school's wires must have gotten crossed when they gave me a woman teacher after spending the year before getting my hands strapped by Mr. B. all the time. I was so comfortable in her class that I took more interest in reading because Mrs. Horne was the assistant librarian, and when Miss Hazel Trembath retired, she would become the new one. Having Mrs. Horne for a teacher was an important event in my life because she got me interested in reading by introducing me to some books that I would be interested in.

Because my family lived so close to the school I went home for lunch every day. I'd have my soup and sandwich and run back to the school to get out on that big field to play sports until the warning bell rang. Terry always took his lunch to school because it would take him too long to walk back and forth.

On November 22, 1963, when I had been back to school for a half hour or so, the school principal came on the public address and told everyone that President Kennedy had been assassinated and we were to go home out of respect for this catastrophe.

Chapter 4
Lose Their Vision

I played catcher in baseball for the same reason I played goal in soccer—so I could play in more games. I started playing sports harder than I'd ever played them before this year because my eagerness to play had turned into an obsession. My willingness to play went into over-drive because I felt that if I proved to the coach that I was a good player I'd be asked to play in each and every game after that. When it was discovered I could slide-check players on the other team to get the ball away from them fairly well, I was moved to a position between defence and forward called halfback. I noticed the guys who played baseball didn't play soccer, and those that played soccer never played baseball. I seemed to be the only one I knew who didn't specialize in playing one sport.

I started thinking of ways I could earn my own money, and when someone mentioned they were a pinsetter at the Port Coquitlam Bowladrome on McAllister Avenue, I decided I wanted to try that. I became a pinsetter and would ride my bike through the underpass and set pins for four or five hours on Saturday mornings for fifteen cents a game. The only dangerous part about the job was making sure I didn't get my legs smacked or my head conked by a pin that unexpectedly went up in the air instead of falling down at the end of the alley. That didn't happen very often but happened when it was least expected. That was the first paying job I had.

I set pins for a few months before I heard about and got a *Vancouver Sun* paper route. That's when *The Sun* still came out in the afternoon instead of the morning. The paper route itself went down to Dominion Avenue to Burns Road when that whole area was still covered with farmland, swamp and bush. I only had about forty-five customers and didn't try for any 'starts' (as delivery people nickered new customers) because I was happy to be out of the house and doing something. Because I was earning my own money, and could afford to buy them, I gave myself permission to start smoking cigarettes. At first I'd always get dizzy, but the more I smoked the quicker my dizzy spells went away whenever I smoked. I knew that if Mom or Dad ever caught me smoking I'd get permanently grounded so I always kept an eye open for them or their friends because I thought they'd tell Mom and Dad if they ever saw me smoking. It only cost twenty-eight cents for a small pack of smokes, and thirty-two for a large deck of cigarettes when I first started smoking. I carried them around in the top of my ginch instead of my shirt or jacket pocket to hide them from the big guys at school. I believed hiding them there would be the best place to hide them because no one would think of looking in someone's underwear for smokes.

Sometimes when it was raining or snowing too much I'd ask Mom or Dad if they would drive me around my paper route because it was too much of a pain to do by bike that day. They usually took pity on me when I asked them and they'd drive me. But most of the time I was out there doing it, six days a week, in all kinds of weather, by myself.

One day, one of my customers put a paper bag with something in it into my paper sack. I thought it was something to eat and planned on eating it later. When I opened the sack, it turned out to be the runt of a litter of kittens. It was the scrawniest thing you ever saw. When I brought the kitten home and the family talked about whether we'd keep it or not, we decided to, and gave it the sarcastic name 'Tiger' because we felt sorry it was the smallest of that litter. In a few short years it was huge. Seeing that cat getting healthier and bigger like it was doing because it was being loved by the family so much, and having it sleep on my bed almost every night turned me into an irreversible cat lover.

GERRY WILLIAMSON

We stopped going to church every Sunday in late 1964; at least I was told I didn't have to keep going to it anymore. That was okay with me because I didn't like having to sit still when I was there, and I couldn't daydream out of the windows because they were made out of stained glass. I had always wondered why we didn't go to church in the summer but had to go the rest of the year.

I spent the 1964-65 school year in a remedial reading class because I believed that Mrs. Horne liked me so much that she wanted to do something to help me become a better reader even if she wasn't my teacher anymore

From October until February I did a *Province* newspaper route (the only early morning newspaper route in this area at that time) as a favour to the son of a family friend because he was the sub-manager of the paper shack (where we got my newspapers from) that have since been replaced by boxes. The route itself was only a few blocks from my house, which was probably why he asked me to do it in the first place. But I had to get the papers from a paper shack on the south side when I was living on the north side of town. It was a good paper route to have even though I didn't like having to get up so early and ride my bike across town because it meant I had to go to bed so early.

The 1964-65 winter had a pretty bad snowfall and when the snow fell as much as it did that year, it upset me physically because it was so hard riding my bike in it. The snow started falling just after I took the route over, and it soon felt worse than the torture of having to get up so early, because I'd get so physically sore. Eventually I was forced to push my bike around the entire route. When that got to be too hard to do I left the bike at home and carried the papers around the route by foot.

I only suspected my grade-six teacher Mrs. B. was one of my customers, but when she answered the door when I was making my first collection it was confirmed.

The only thing I liked about all that snow was going bumper riding once in a while, which is grabbing onto the rear bumper of a car and letting it pull you behind it. Doing that was fun, but it could be hard on a bumper-rider too, especially when the snow was melting and parts

34

of the road were showing. When I'd hit a spot on the road that didn't have any compact snow on it, I'd wipe out all over the place. I didn't get the strap from the principal all year in grade six because I didn't fool around in class because I was too busy learning how to read. But weekends were different. That's when most of my mischievous character defects woke up.

I'd met a guy named Gord when I was still doing my *Vancouver Sun* paper route and we started hanging out together at that time because the border between his route and mine rubbed shoulders with each other (they were beside each other) so we saw each other almost every day. One Sunday, Gord and I decided to get into some perfectly good trouble by writing graffiti on every single door of Viscount because we had the time to kill that day. It only took us about two hours to do it all because we were more diligent about finishing this self-gratifying task than anything we'd ever done before. The only reason we got caught was because Gord never washed the blue felt-pen ink off his hands, and the only reason I didn't get caught as his accomplice was because Gord never finked on me by telling the principal I'd told him how to spell all the big words.

None of the staff at the school had ever seen us together before no one knew we'd once had paper routes so close together and we never hung out together at school because we were in different classes. Gord and I weren't allowed to be friends after that because his dad considered me incorrigible. Since that word sounded so nifty to me I thought it was neat being called that. I looked the word up in the dictionary when I became older and it told me that it means uncontrollable, unruly, and unmanageable—Oops.

Seeing Terry physically worsening caused Mom and Dad to accept the fact that there was a bigger problem with him than they had originally thought. From that mustard-seed size of acceptance, question marks started dancing in their minds and they consulted a different doctor for a different diagnosis because they had both convinced themselves that our family doctor at that time put more faith in what a man said than what a woman thought, so Mom made all the arrangements for Dad to take Terry to see a specialist because they both knew the day-to-day challenges of raising Terry while the family doctor was only looking at the problem clinically.

This specialist told Dad the same thing that a different family doctor had told Mom and Dad years earlier—that 'Terry would outgrow this stage of his life.' And because Mom and Dad had already anticipated hearing him say these words, Dad had the specialist watch how Terry did stairs before giving his final answer. Terry had always gone up the stairs on all fours and come down them on his bum because it was easier for him to do it that way. When the specialist saw him doing this, he stopped believing what he thought was true and accepted what he saw was the truth.

Terry was put in the hospital to have tests and experiments performed on him. The final analysis would involve the removal of a portion of muscle tissue taken from the back of his calf and the side of his arm to be examined under a microscope.

When Dad went to the hospital to pick Terry up in another week he had to physically carry him to the car. When they were a few blocks from home, as a joke, Terry told Dad to tell everyone in the family that the hospital decided to keep him for a while and scrunched down on the floor in the back seat. When Mom went to the car to get something a few minutes later, Terry appeared yelling, 'Surprise.' As Mom told me this in 1998, her eyes clouded with tears.

I was under the strict impression that Terry couldn't walk at that time because his scars hadn't healed yet. I think Terry wanted to believe that he'd be getting better soon too, because for the next few years he was always saying to me, 'When I start riding my bike again I'm going to…' or he'd say, 'When I start walking again I'm…'

It was years before he stopped talking about riding his bike and walking again. I thought he was only going to be in that wheelchair that Mom and Dad got for him until he got over his operation. But, as time slipped into the past faster than anticipated, I realized differently.

Our whole family already knew that once Terry's brain grabbed onto anything for any length of time, that thing was never released into forgetfulness. For example, one time after the family had gone to my aunt and uncle's house in the United States one time before, Terry was telling us when we'd be hitting all the little bumps and dips on the road long before we got to where they were, and he'd also be telling us where and when we were supposed to be turning—like he was reading a map. I didn't want to believe he had a photographic memory at that time, but his mind seemed to be getting stronger as his body was getting weaker—the same way a blind person's hearing improves as they lose their vision.

Chapter 5
In the Hospital

At first, Viscount didn't want Terry returning after his operation because they didn't think the school would be suitable for someone in a wheelchair. Mom raised so much stink about this that Terry was reinstated in September 1965 and I began pushing him back and forth to school every day. Jackie started going to an all-girls private school in New Westminster called St. Ann's Academy (no longer there), for her grade-eleven year.

I wanted to become a bagpiper and joined the 72nd Seaforth Highlanders on Burrard Street in Vancouver to do this. But I erased my plans to become a piper when the bagpipe instructor (a friend of Mom and Dad's) told them I'd have to learn how to play a type of flute called a chanter first. I decided to stay in cadets anyway because it got me out of the house one day out of the week.

Usually there were three of us cadets picked up by an army truck at the Commercial Hotel (where Shaughnessy Square is today—on the corner of Flint and Lougheed) every Wednesday night at 7:30 and taken into the Seaforth Armoury and returned at 10:30.

At the start of my last year of elementary school I was presented with another man teacher who enjoyed smacking kids on the hands as much as my grade-four teacher had. Mr. C. must have appreciated my behaviour because he had me stand in front of him when we were getting this class picture taken.

He also demonstrated how much he appreciated me by having me sit in the front row of the class soon after the school year began so he could keep an eye on me all the time. In the past I'd start most school years off by sitting near the back of the room, and by the time we got our first report card I'd be sitting in the first row.

There was a girl in that class that I didn't become friends with at that time because I thought she was trying to be the 'teacher's pet' by choice, and I was afraid this imagined attitude of mine would rub off on me if I was friends with her, because whenever Mr. C. left the room she was always put in charge of the class. It turns out she hated this. Again I was the first in the class to get whacked across the hands because I was more interested in entertaining the rest of the class when I should have been listening to him. He mentioned this when he wrote this on my first report card of the year, 'Gerry is trying to be the "class buffoon."'

For some reason everybody in the family thought that was one of the worst things a teacher could say about me. They had good reason to think that because I was getting my hands smacked almost every day at school for something I'd done—sometimes I got it two or three times a day. I still wanted to show Mom and Dad that I wasn't the class buffoon, and did my best to master grade seven because I knew I could still do two things at once without too much trouble. Still, there were things I learned while pretending I wasn't paying attention to what was going on.

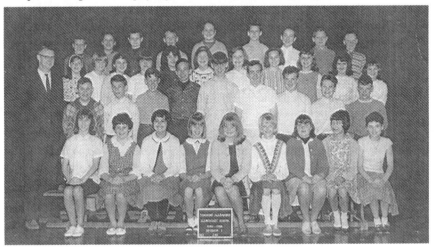

**Grade seven class at Viscount—
I'm in the second row—first on the left**

39

For the summer of 1966 Mom and Dad rented a trailer for us to use when we went on holidays because it was probably going to be the last time the entire family could go on a vacation together, because Jackie was going to graduate from high school in June and might not be able to have holidays at the same time as Mom and Dad had theirs next summer. They also wanted to see how we liked using a trailer because it would be ideal for Terry.

After spending a relaxing two weeks with relatives in BC's interior, and we were all relaxed and feeling tired on our way home with Dad driving the car and trailer and with Mom acting as his co-pilot in the front seat and Jackie and me riding in the back seat. Terry was in his usual spot (the big open area at the back of the station wagon.)

After coming down a long hill before starting on a straight stretch going into Grand Forks, the car and trailer suddenly dove over an embankment between two telephone poles—landing on the edge of a farmer's field with a plop instead of a crash. We were immediately forced into a moment of silence, not realizing that something had just happened for about three seconds; no one recognized that we'd just survived a potentially fatal accident, no one understood that a few seconds ago we were speeding along the highway and the next we were doing zero beside it. When that moment of silence ended and everyone was recognizing that something had just happened to us, Terry was more concerned about everyone else's welfare than about his own.

He seemed to do everything that way because he could. While I, on the other hand, was far too busy barrelling through my life knocking things down that were in the way because I could, sat there in shock.

Meanwhile cars had pulled off to the side of the road with the passengers looking over the embankment expecting to see—because of where the accident happened—a car full of fatalities down the hill. When they saw Terry's wheelchair in the back of the station wagon, for some reason their eyes shone like they'd hit pay dirt. Dad never drove the car with more than one other family member in it again.

When we got home in a couple of days I didn't think about my close shave with death because I didn't think it was such a big deal.

I'd met Gord's cousin, Ken, when he took over Gord's paper route. And when I was told I couldn't be friends with Gord anymore I started hanging out with him because we got along so well. I always made sure I stayed away from Ken's place whenever Gord's parents were visiting Ken's folks because I thought Gord's dad thought I was a hopeless goofball by thinking I had enough power to talk Gord into doing all that writing on the doors at Viscount.

Terry was a special person, but I failed to recognize this at the time because he was my brother, in the same way that the people of Galilee didn't think Jesus was anyone special either because everybody in that area knew him.

He turned out to have the most severe childhood form of muscular dystrophy called Duchene dystrophy—where the age of onset and its severity vary from person to person and the disease progresses steadily without remission. It occurs only in boys.

His schooling at Viscount came to an end when some cruel-minded, future criminal types took his good nature as a sign of weakness and pushed him into a ditch and left him there. Mom had to go to the school and pick him up. That ended my having to push Terry to school.

Because society didn't know how to deal with people with the kinds of problems Terry had, these confused parts were hid in plain sight with other people with similar problems. I don't remember being told why he had to go to a different school at the time, but suddenly every school morning, a bunny-bus (a van converted to carry people in wheelchairs) would arrive in our driveway to take him to a special school.

Going to that school ended when Mom and Dad discovered that Terry wasn't learning anything there because he would usually end up helping the teacher take care of the other kids in the classroom because of what their illnesses were doing to them. A more suitable school was needed, so names of places were bounced back and forth until Sunny Hill Hospital for Children in Vancouver was chosen. Terry would be living in this hospital during the week and coming home for the weekend because his mind was like any other muscle in the human body—he had to use it or he'd lose it.

Mom and Dad said we were moving to a house we were having built that had a ground-floor basement. When we moved into this house we started carrying Terry upstairs all the time in his wheelchair for his meals, but after doing this a few times someone figured out that it would be easier on Terry's nerves and our muscles to bring his meals down to him. Instead of putting Terry into solitary confinement at meal times, he and I could eat our dinner while watching TV together. This eventually made me feel I wasn't part of the family on the weekend, the same way Terry might have felt he wasn't part of the family the rest of the week while he was in the hospital.

Chapter 6
In Common With

The 1966-67 school year was my first year of high school and Jackie's last year of school. She had already decided to go back to PoCo so she could graduate with the people she started high school with. She'd also warned me that juniors (which I'd be) weren't allowed to talk to seniors (which she'd be) or they'd get a 'detention' (DT) and would have to sit in the detention room (a designated room where all the students who got DT's that day went to after school and sat with their hands behind their back for thirty-five minutes.) That didn't sound like a lot of fun to me, and because she looked so serious when she was telling me this I believed her, and made it a point to stay away from her as much as possible at school.

The first time I walked into PoCo the very first person I saw was a beautiful long-dark-haired girl I later found out was named Louise. I was freaked out I was going to the same school as someone so attractive! After a few days of going to high school I noticed other juniors talking to seniors all the time, and because I didn't care if I talked to Jackie at school or not, I became blind whenever I saw her in the hallway. I've since figured out that the only reason she told me such a Technicolor lie like that was because I always seemed to do something that embarrassed her in playing my role as her little brother so well. I still had a lot of Grade-A good times in grade eight that Jackie didn't acknowledge or know about. At least, if she did, she didn't mention them to Mom and Dad. One reason she might not have told them about all the fooling around I did was because I was never called to the principal's office over PoCo's PA, but was sent directly there so everybody in the school didn't know I'd been summoned. I was far from being an angel though; I either instigated or took part in different disturbances around the school: I was in a short pie fight in the cafeteria, I put banana peels on the floor outside of classrooms to see if anyone would slip on them (no one did,) I threw snowballs in the halls. I did anything I thought was funny. One time almost everyone in my Music 8 class threw chewed-to-a-pulp pieces of paper against almost the entire ceiling of the music room. These wads managed to stick surprisingly well.

Then there was the time that a friend of mine named Pat talked another friend of mine I nickered Little Billy and me into having a mock boxing match in the gymnasium in front of everyone who would pay to see it one lunch hour. We only wanted to charge the other students a dime to watch it, so they couldn't afford not to see it. I didn't have anything to do with the organizing of the event because I didn't think it was going to happen, but when I started seeing posters adverting it on the walls I realized that it was too late to back out of now.

When the big day for the boxing match arrived I treated it like it was happening to someone else, because I thought I was one of those people who satisfied themselves by watching things happen instead of making things happen. In fact, I'd always been one of those people who caused so much havoc to happen around them, that they couldn't see they'd caused it in the first place.

I didn't think this fight was going to be such a big deal until we walked into the gym and I saw the bleachers were full of people. We raised over $50 for the Gerald Daniel's Fund (an African boy the school had adopted) to watch me lose.

Near the end of the school year Mom and Dad were so upset with me for doing so lousy at school that they threatened to enrol me in a private all-boys Catholic school in Burnaby called St. Thomas More. I didn't want to go there because I would have to wear a shirt and tie and would have to make all new friends. To show Mom and Dad that I could change myself without having to be enrolled in STM I decided to go to army cadet camp.

Another reason I wanted to go to cadet camp was because it was the only way to be promoted in cadets, other than by staying in them for years and years, and I wanted to be promoted to a sergeant so badly that I could almost feel the three stripes being sewn on the right sleeve of my tunic.

I'd waited too long to sign up for the Cadet Leader Program, which all future NCO's or non-commissioned officers have to take before being promoted. I'd procrastinated about signing up for camp until the only thing left to take was band. I didn't know how to play a musical instrument or anything, but signed up for it anyway because I didn't expect to be allowed to go.

To prepare me for going to army camp Mom told me her version of 'the facts of life' by saying, "You know that thing between your legs?" I nodded yes. "Well, it's not just for peeing out of you know. I want you to treat every girl like she was your sister," she concluded. Those few words caused all sorts of scaredy-cats to explode into serious phobias in my mind that I forced myself to remember forever.

Dad told me his version of 'the facts' and they were, "You'll be lucky to have two people in your entire life you can count on as a true friend." And "Once you hit twenty the years are going to speed by you faster than you ever thought they would." I laughed at that because I was sixteen at the time and I had tons of what I considered to be good friends. I've since figured out that the only reason time was moving so slow at that time was because I didn't have a very long past to compare it to. That wasn't the first nor the last time I'd confused quantity with quality in my life either. I've since lived long enough to know that what Dad was telling me was the truth.

Neither Mom nor Dad ever came out and said what I was about to hear was going to be 'the facts of life,' but I assumed that's what they were. I always thought they were going to be about sex, but they were about how to live life instead.

It had been a long-standing tradition of the cadets who had already been to camp to tell the cadets going there for their first time to ask the commanding officer for their 'masturbation papers' before going to camp. I knew what that word meant and never had to ask. I'd also heard about the bad apples of the barracks being held down and having handfuls of black shoe polish smeared on their genitals. I was worried that something like that would happen to me, but I became confident I wasn't going to get black-balled because I decided not to fool around at camp all summer.

After we got to camp and were issued the khaki-coloured short pants and short-sleeved shirts that we'd be wearing all summer and getting the instruments we'd be playing for the rest of the summer too, I saw that the only instrument that didn't look too hard to play was the bass drum. Without giving it much thought I decided I wanted to play that because I'd be noticed more. But I was given a tenor drum instead because there already was someone at camp that played the bass drum in a marching band in his corps.

When we first started having band practice I learned that all I had to do was watch the other tenor drummer and do what he did. That's how I learned to play tenor drum.

I'd never been away from everyone in my family on my birthday before, so when Mom was visiting relatives in the Okanogan she took Jackie, Terry, and me out for my birthday supper. We met a cousin of mine at a restaurant outside of Vernon, and halfway through the meal the corporal in charge of the barracks I slept in walked in. I was hoping he'd come over to the table and say something to me so I could show off for everyone in the family, but he didn't.

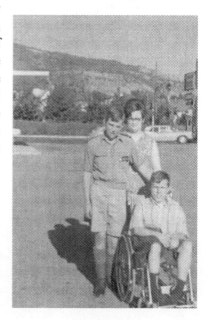

Cadet Williamson with Jackie and Terry at Vernon Army Cadet camp on July 10, 1967.

There was a guy at camp that I knew from the 72nd who had been to camp a few times before. He stayed in a different barracks than me, but we'd always get together in our off hours and walk to Polson Park and hang out together there. One Sunday after lunch we walked into a field and climbed into a long wooden trough called a flume (used for carrying water to the fields for irrigation.) The water in this aqueduct traveled fast enough to carry us a long way before we had to get out of the water and walk back to where we started from. The weather was so hot in that part of the province at that time of the year that our clothes were desert dry by the time we got back in the water to go again.

When I was away at camp I had tried sniffing gasoline, nail-polish remover and airplane glue a few times, but found the high I got from them didn't last very long. And every time I smoked dope I'd get paranoid and figured that those paranoid feelings were the high I was supposed to get and decided I didn't need drugs to make me feel the way I didn't like feeling and left drugs alone because they made me feel things I didn't like feeling. So I switched over to drinking booze instead, because I thought everyone I knew was doing the same thing. I thought I had to use something unnatural to make myself feel natural.

Now that Jackie had graduated from high school I decided to stick my finger into the pie of the sixties and see what I pulled out. I felt the freedom to experiment in the newer things happening around the school without having to worry about her finking out on me all the time.

When we were picking out our locker partners for the grade-nine high school year, everybody in my homeroom class had already picked someone to be their locker partner except another guy, a girl and me. I quickly asked the attractive girl to be my partner because I was jealous the other guy would ask her to be his partner before I did. Having Susan for a locker partner helped me want to change the way I was with other people.

I still wasn't through with being a kid though, and one Saturday in late September Ken and I walked to Minnekhada Ranch (now Lodge) because we heard there were some trout farms behind them. We weren't planning on doing any damage or anything; we just wanted to see if the story we heard was true. We were successful in sneaking onto the property easy enough, and when we found the ponds we saw we couldn't see any fish in them because the pools were in the shade. We decided to leave before we were caught, but before we got very far along the trail we spotted a guy who looked like he was looking for us. So we jumped into a creek and stood in the glacier-cold water waiting for the guy to leave. The guy must have seen us jumping into the creek because he walked right over to the bridge we were hiding under and waited on it for us to start feeling stupid for standing in ice water. The scenario that started playing in my mind told me that this guy knew we were hiding under that bridge and was willing to wait on it for us to start feeling wacky-bananas for standing in the water.

I finally got tired of waiting for him to leave, before he got tired of waiting for us to get out of the water, and decided to turn myself in. Ken followed my lead. The guy wanted our parents' phone numbers, so we gave them to him. I was lucky he phoned Ken's place before he phoned mine because my folks never found out about what happened that day.

When Ken's dad came and picked us up he told us we weren't allowed to have contact with each other for six months. We obeyed this order until one day I decided to go over to Ken's place when his parents were out, and I was still there when they pulled into the driveway before we expected them. This threw me into a state of momentary confusion because I didn't know what door they'd use to enter the house, and I knew I'd be in trouble up to my arm-pits if I was caught inside the house. Without thinking about what I was doing I jumped out Ken's second-story bedroom window and landed on their cement driveway and ran home the instant they walked in the house.

I had signed up for Typing 9 near the end of grade eight because my handwriting was so lousy (still is) and there was an old typewriter at home that no one seemed to be using that I'd sometimes use the trusted 'H and P' (Hunt & Peck) method on when writing paragraphs, essays and book reports to get a higher mark. I thought if I learned where all the letters were it wouldn't take me as long to type what I was writing. My typing speed only got up to about twenty words a minute, but I learned where all the letters were. I'd also signed up for Metalwork 9 because I heard you could sneak a smoke in the metalwork shop if the forge was turned on. I only had about four smokes there all year, so taking the class didn't balance itself out to the amount of smokes I had. But I did learn that cigarette smoke goes up the fan system when it was turned on because cigarette smoke is attracted by heat or something like that. From learning that, I figured out that if I rolled some newspapers up and set them on fire and stuck them up the chimney I could get a flow of hot air moving from the fireplace and out of the house.

I felt that I'd grown up a lot because I'd been to cadet camp and because I wanted to change the way I looked to girls, I understood I had to slim down a lot. I knew I would have to make changes in the way I ate or I would never lose any weight. In order to do that, my common sense told me I'd have to stop eating the way I'd always eaten, which was eating whatever I wanted to eat, whenever I wanted to eat it. I also knew I couldn't lose any weight by thinking it away and decided to start playing organized sports again in order to burn off some calories.

There were no football, soccer or baseball teams at PoCo, and I didn't like playing basketball. The only other sport left to play was rugby and I didn't have a clue how to play that. For those readers who don't know anything about rugby, like I didn't, I'll give you a short-cut version of it. It's sort of like American football but it's not as dainty because you don't wear all those protective pads that football players wear. As a result you get hurt a lot more, which I didn't think would happen to me.

I always got a belly full of scaredy-cats when showing up for my first try-out of any sport. We weeded ourselves off the team if we felt we couldn't take (hack) the punishment of playing rugby after a while. At first, the junior rugby coach hardly let me play in the games at all, and the times he did let me play were the last few minutes of the game when it was assured our team would win or lose. I thought that the coach was keeping me on the team to make the other players look better at that time.

The first season I played rugby, I hardly played in the games themselves, but was told to run lines, which is running along the side-lines of the field the game was being played on to let the referee know where the ball had gone out of bounds, so he'd know where to throw the ball back into play. This would cause the players to have a lineout, where members of each team's scrum (the brute force, and one of the most important aspects of the game) would line up beside each other perpendicular into the playing field and jump for the ball that a 'wing' has thrown between the rows of opposing players.

There were two seasons of rugby each school year; from mid-September to mid-December, and from mid-February to mid-May. I decided I wasn't going to play anymore because I wasn't given the chance to learn how to play. But from all those lines I'd run, I saw I was losing weight and becoming a faster runner. When I realized that, it dawned on me that I might be a good rugby player one of these days and decided to keep playing.

As time tick-tocked itself into my second season I was being asked to play in more and more games. I eventually lost a lot of baby fat in three months on that egg-and-grapefruit diet that I put myself on. Which for me was eating two poached eggs on dry toast, followed by an entire grapefruit for breakfast, and the same thing for lunch, and then a normal supper.

Ken and I were hardly seeing each other at school anymore, so I started hanging out with other people. This started me thinking of looking for a new best friend that I had more in common with.

Chapter 7
Time Not Thinking

The first time I met Skip was in April 1968 when my Socials Studies 9 teacher, Mr. Moore (who had also been my rugby coach when I first started playing junior rugby), introduced him to the class by saying, "Everyone, this is a new student, named Skip." I quickly said, "Skip a rope" and the entire class exploded into a mess of laughter. I was immediately given a DT of cleaning the doodles off of desks after school because of my spontaneity. We saw each other around the school a few times after that and that was it.

But on New Year's Eve day in 1969 after I'd drank a concoction that I called Swampwater (made from pouring a few ounces out of every bottle of booze Mom and Dad had in their liquor cabinet into a beer bottle) along the way to Skip's house with Ken, I started thinking that things would never work out for Ken and me because of the strain on our friendship by his dad. I was smoking my pipe to hide my boozy breath when I got to Skip's house and I remember Skip's dad coming up to within a breath-smelling distance of my face and asking me if I was allowed to smoke that pipe at home. I said I was. In fact smoking that pipe in front of Mom and Dad was the first step to smoking cigarettes in front of them because I knew they would know a pipe smoker doesn't inhale and they'd let me smoke a pipe because of that. I also knew that if I were allowed to smoke a pipe in front of them it wouldn't take that much persuasion to get them to let me smoke cigarettes in front of them in the future.

Skip told me he was a Queen Scout, which didn't mean that much to me at the time, because I didn't know that becoming one was so hard to do when you're as young as he was. All three of my Aunty Wava's sons, Dave, Rick and Jim, were Queen Scouts but that's all I knew about Queen Scouts. Skip showed me his uniform with all his earned badges sewn neatly on the sleeves. He had so many it looked like both arms were nothing but badges. Seeing this made me feel internally embarrassed that I'd only earned a single Collector's Badge when I was in cubs.

Due to the fact that football and rugby are similar in tackling and roughness I asked Skip if he wanted to play rugby because he once told me he enjoyed playing football. When rugby season started in January 1969 he came with me to join the team. Skip was asked to play in the three-line, which is made up of the fastest running and most agile players on the team, the first time he came out to play. I felt a little embarrassed by this, because it was my third season of playing rugby and I was still playing in the scrum when I wanted to be playing in the three-line. I decided to start playing rugby harder than I'd ever played it before because I knew all I needed to do was add 'the try and improve' part to myself and I'd improve as a player.

Because my rugby playing had improved so much after running all those lines and losing all that weight I stopped thinking the coach was keeping me on the team to make the other players look better, and I started believing he was letting me play more because I was getting better and better.

One time, after Skip and I had established ourselves as friends, I brought a bottle of cheap wine over to his house and started drinking it. After I drank about half of it I started puking in his bathroom downstairs; meanwhile his brother, Kim, had found my bottle and had a few healthy belts out of it was barfing in the can upstairs.

I was finding that I was getting drunk fast and thought I was just too young to drink, so that October I started going to what I called 'pop and chip parties' with Skip and about ten or twelve other people at different people's houses every second weekend because I didn't want to drink because I was a lousy drinker. At these parties we'd drink punch and eat potato chips and dance all night long. In late November I first heard **The BEATLES** album for the first time and fell in love with music, especially Beatles music, after that.

I felt I'd worked hard to get into such good physical condition and deserved a little more attention than I was getting from everyone at home. But no one there seemed to focus any on me. This lack of attention made me determined to become an even better rugby player than I'd ever imagined I'd be at this time.

By the time I was very far into my third rugby season I was moved from playing in the scrum to playing left wing at the end of the three-line—I was the guy who threw the ball back into play in line-outs. I noticed that most of the guys who were good at playing soccer and touch football in elementary school never played rugby in high school, but preferred playing basketball instead.

I had flunked both math and French in grade nine and Mom insisted I stay on the academic/technical program in grade ten because she'd always known my mind worked as fast as it did and I was only pretending to be dumb in school. But I wasn't aware of that at that time because I had thoroughly confused myself into believing I was either a part-time genius or a bit of a loony-tune years before. Time pushed the boy in me out of the window of junior rugby into the rough-tough scaredy-cat world of senior rugby in my last two years of high school. I'd already created this mystique about senior rugby in my mind that told me all the players on that team were rough and tough. The senior boys rugby coach (Mr. Marsden) must have seen me playing wing in junior rugby and thought I was a pretty good team player (even though I wasn't a high scorer because he kept me a winger on his team).

I'd improved as a rugby player so much that I played in every game for the entire game until I finished high school after that. I wore a number two on the back of my jersey which didn't mean I was the second best player on the team, it just meant my jersey had a number two on the back of it. Strange as coincidences sometimes are, number two is my lucky number.

In senior rugby we started each practice off by running two or three laps around the track to get warmed up, and then the actual practices started where we'd do a bunch of sit-ups, push-ups and dive-outs—running as hard as we could and diving straight ahead onto the frozen or muddy ground while giving a killer-diller scream (while in the air) about ten or fifteen times. Then we'd line up in two rows and someone in one of the lines would start running and someone in the other line would tackle them. After that, we'd change sides and the other guy would do the tackling. We ended each practice by running more laps around the track.

About halfway through my first season of senior rugby when we were playing a home game I dove for a bouncing ball when someone on the other team decided to boot it. I took the full force of the kick in the face. I played for another ten or fifteen minutes, but every time I ran my nose kept flopping from one side of my face to the other and I had to quit playing because just taking the pain wasn't doing the trick for me. I went into RCH a couple of days later and had my nose repaired. Gauze was stuffed up my left nostril and it stayed in there for about a week. When the nose was set enough, the doctor grabbed the exposed end of the wadding with tweezers and yanked it out. I felt a little tingling feeling inside my nose, and then blood started flowing out of it and he had to cauterize it to stop the bleeding. Every time I feel that same feeling today I know my nose is going to start bleeding. Once you've experienced a feeling like that, it's impossible to forget—it will remain with me along with all the other first-time feelings I've felt in life already—like the first bottle of beer I ever drank, the first inhaled cigarette and the first romantic kiss I ever had, etc.

Terry always told me his feet got cold at night, so I got into the habit of leaving his socks on him when putting him to bed for the night. His lower extremities probably weren't getting warmed up enough sitting in his wheelchair all the time. He also knew what time we'd be picking him up at Sunny Hill every Friday night and would be waiting for us by the front door of the hospital. The times I went with Mom or Dad to pick him up and he wasn't waiting by the front door I'd stay in the car and let them go in and get him because I had created a scaredy-cat in my mind that told me I might catch whatever the other patients there had.

Terry was so happy-go-lucky and remembered everyone's name so effortlessly that he made friends with everyone he met. All he had to do was be himself and he'd draw people to him like a magnet attracts metal. Nobody felt they had to act the way perfectly good strangers acted with other perfectly good strangers with him because he was the same with everybody. Terry loved drinking beer and he was always telling me he couldn't wait until he was twenty-one (the drinking age in BC at that time) when the two of us could go to the Commercial Hotel and have a few glasses of beer together. I kept this memory alive by not forgetting it.

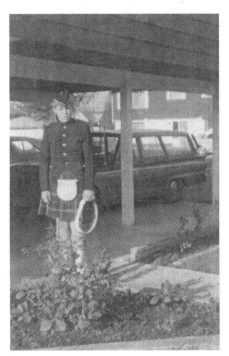

Dress Blues in 1968.

When I'd gone back to school in 1970 I decided not to return to cadets because I wanted to grow my hair longer. I also decided I was going to change myself the same way I'd changed myself when I went to cadet camp.

It seemed like Mom and Dad had taken it for granted that I wanted to stay home with Terry when I didn't go to these 'pop and chip parties.' They never came right out and said I had to stay home with him, it just seemed like they took it for granted that I wanted to, because no one told me I didn't have to.

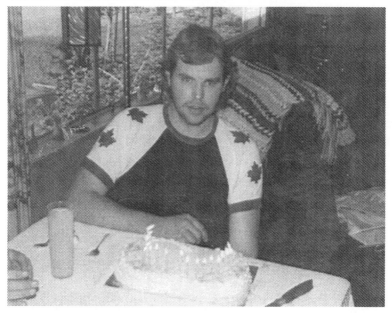

My 17th Birthday in July 1969.

To me it seemed that Terry always copied everything I did when we were together because it appeared like he was so proud I could do what he couldn't. He joined an Air Cadet squadron in Burnaby at this time. That is what gave me the impression he was pretending we were living the same adventure in life; like whenever I cut someone else down (belittled them) he'd immediately be on my side belittling that same person.

Sometimes I thought Terry didn't even know who the person I was cutting down was! I didn't realize that he was flattering me at the time he was doing that.

One day around my seventeenth birthday Skip told me he had to live off the land for a couple of days to become a Queen Scout. And because I wanted to experience the same things as him, we decided to hike up Burke Mountain and go to Munroe Lake and live off the land in late July 1969. We spent hours and hours hiking up there and I was looking forward to swimming in a beautiful lake when we arrived, but all we found when we got there was a stagnant pond. I felt so disappointed about this that I decided I should drink the bottle of Swampwater I'd brought along. Then we caught a bunch of tadpoles and cooked them and were considering eating them but chickened out at the last second and ate a huge bowl of nothing instead!

This adventure was supposed to be stamped with a gold seal of first-class approval as being one of the highlights of the summer for us, but it was turning into one of the worst experiences of our lives. There we were in our sleeping bags at 4:00 p.m. trying to escape the millions of mosquitoes trying to eat us alive and having a small-talk chitchat when one of us remembered hearing on the radio that the US was going to be landing a man on the moon for the first time the next day.

That would be the high point of the summer for anyone because space flights were still a novelty at that time. In fact that would be one of the biggest big deals to happen to anyone as far as history-making events were concerned. We couldn't miss that, could we?

When the next morning woke us up we walked over to Coast Meridian and started the long walk home. Part of the way down the hill I decided we should keep walking to the Northside Shopping Centre and go to Young's Pharmacy (since moved and two stores were combined into making a neighbourhood pub at that location) and get something to eat. Once we'd gotten to Young's we bought some of the goodies I'd been daydreaming about eating all weekend long to stave off some of the hunger I was feeling before going to my house to watch the event on TV.

We did that, and when we opened the basement door to the house Terry yelled out from the rumpus room, "You missed them taking the first step on the moon by five minutes." That pleased us black and blue because if we hadn't gone for something to eat we would have heard the first word said by a human on the moon, "Contact lights. Houston, the Eagle has landed." And seeing Neil Armstrong taking that 'one small step for man' live. Missing him taking that 'giant leap for mankind' was the first time I became aware that there were lots of once-in-a-lifetime events I was missing out on because I was spending too much time not thinking.

Chapter 8
Broken Fingers

The camaraderie amongst us rugby players was so strong that I started going to as many bush and house parties on weekends as possible. This contributed to me trying too hard to have a good time at these parties. I was getting drunk more and more, because in my mind rugby playing and beer drinking went together. I also thought that because I was a rugby player it was expected that I wanted to be a beer drinker and be 'wild and crazy' more than other people.

It didn't take long before I became an accident looking for somewhere to happen. Mom and Dad wanted to stop me from having that accident, and when the summer of 1970 was about to take place they made arrangements for me to go to Uranium City, Saskatchewan, to spend the summer with Go and his wife, Tina. Go came to Port Coquitlam to pick me up and we flew to Edmonton and changed planes to fly the rest of the way into Eldorado, which was a short distance away from his house in Uranium City. From the air the town looked like a handful of Monopoly houses were planted there. After I'd arrived, Go took me to the Uranium City Bakery and asked the owner if I could work there for the rest of the summer to give his full-time employee the rest of the summer off. The owner said I could, and I learned the art of being a baker's assistant.

One of the first things I had to learn when I was up north was how to sleep when it was still light outside. We were so far north that it was light outside the entire summer. It wasn't bright sunshine at midnight or anything, but you could easily see.

I spent one Sunday going into the wilds of Northern Saskatchewan on a canoe trip with some of Go and Tina's friends. We had to portage the canoe that we'd borrowed from a Chippewa Indian quite a few times over beaver dams.

The BC government lowered the drinking age from twenty-one to nineteen on July 1, 1970. I thought that because the drinking age was lowered I had to drink when I became nineteen because I believed I'd be able to drink better then.

Go and Tina and I went to where Go worked and I saw the procedure of refining uranium ore into pure uranium. There were these huge tumblers with big metal balls bouncing around inside them to crush the ore. The actual refined uranium was a brighter shade of yellow than sulphur. Even with the amount of dust floating in the air the workers didn't wear masks or any other protective clothing.

I spent hours and hours writing long rambling letters to different people after the novelty of being up north had worn off. I found I enjoyed writing these letters but considered writing them to be the solution to the boredom I was feeling. I really enjoyed writing these letters and thought briefly of becoming a journalist when I finished with high school, but all I did with that thought was think about it. Another thing I did to relieve the boredom I was feeling was going to the movies by myself because the only people I knew there were Go and Tina's friends, and they were all in their twenties or older and I didn't think they wanted to be my friend.

There was a university-attending girl who had gone on the canoe trip, that I'd often see taking the tickets when I went to see the movies. She was a year or two older than me and because she was so much older I didn't think she would be interested in me.

When I flew back to Edmonton at the end of August to catch a flight back to Vancouver, there was a three-hour lay-over there so I did some window-shopping and bought *The Beatles Illustrated Lyrics* by Alan Aldridge, and some love beads.

Being up north like that was the first time I discovered I could spend most of my time by myself and it wouldn't bother me. Sometimes I liked being alone better. I also found out there is a huge difference between being alone in solitude and feeling alone in loneliness.

A lot had changed about me during the summer that I hadn't realized at first. The biggest change was probably my body. I was now a powerful machine from doing bakers' work all summer so I felt excited about going back to PoCo after working up north for those two months because I realized I'd just had a once-in-a-lifetime adventure that I would never forget.

My desire to be cool came alive this year, and to make myself feel sweet I started wearing those love beads I'd bought in Edmonton all the time.

My last year of high school was the first year of the semester system for the students going to PoCo. So, after I had my classes assigned to me I knew the last half of the year would pass quickly because all my hard classes were in the first semester.

In October 1970, Mom and Dad gave me the money to buy a blue leather rugby jacket with PORT COQUITLAM RUGBY CLUB sewn on the front of it, and number two sewn on the right sleeve. The championship crest the rugby team had won in Junior Rugby was sewn on the left sleeve too. I started wearing that jacket everywhere at school to make sure everybody who saw me knew I played on a championship rugby team.

Skip asked me if I wanted to join an organization that was a step above Scouts called Venturers. I didn't want to join at first because it seemed I had just gotten out of cadets a few years before, and I had only been in cubs for a year, many years before that, but I went with him anyway because that's what friends do.

One time a group of us went to where the group leader worked in the Gastown section of Vancouver, and we saw an entire room full of equipment that was one single computer. I never thought computers would ever add up to anything important in the future because all I saw them do at that time was make pictures with letters and numbers. When I mentioned this to Dad he told me that one of these days computers would run absolutely everything. I didn't want to believe him because I was older than sixteen, and as anyone who has lived past sixteen has already found out for themselves, some sixteen-year-old guys think they are experts on things they haven't experienced yet.

Mom and Dad let me smoke cigarettes in front of them. Maybe they let me smoke because they thought that smoking wasn't hurting them any and it wouldn't hurt Jackie and me either. Jackie didn't inhale, but I made up for her. Now that I was allowed to smoke at home I started feeling like how I thought a grown-up felt. The thrill of getting caught smoking was now gone and I started feeling like I wouldn't be treated like a kid that much longer.

I don't think Terry was as happy at home as he was at Sunny Hill because he was left alone so much at home. He eased the fears and frustrations of a lot of the newer people to the hospital by being himself. He had the unofficial but important job of making the newer kids to the hospital feel more comfortable about being away from home for perhaps the first time in their lives.

He'd been institutionalized from living in Sunny Hill for so long that an internal alarm clock went off in his head that woke him up early in the morning. Once he was awake, it seemed he expected me to be as eager beaver to greet the new day as he was. He was probably so eager to greet the new day because he had waited all week to come home for the weekend and I wasn't as excited about being at home as he was because I was there all the time.

Because I've always felt that weekends were a time to sleep in, that's exactly what I wanted to do. But early every Saturday and Sunday morning I'd always hear Terry's voice whispering my name over and over, "Gerry Gerry Gerry Gerry Gerry Gerry Gerry Gerry Gerry Gerry Gerry Gerry Gerry Gerry," until I'd feel guilty about not being up and felt compelled to get out of bed, get him dressed and into his wheelchair and out the bedroom door. After I'd gotten him up, I was always left wide-awake because I'd just concentrated so much on doing what I had to do to get him up. From years of doing this I knew it was pointless to try and go back to sleep again.

One time Skip and I decided we'd try smoking some marijuana, but the pot we'd bought had been cured in something that Skip's brain reacted to, and made him go funny in the sanity department for a while. I became closer to his mom at this time when I found out that grown-ups weren't the enemy as I had always thought grown-ups were. That was the last time I allowed anyone to see me cry like a baby, because when Skip was sleeping off the effects of the drugs downstairs in his bedroom, I was upstairs bawling like a baby with his mom because I felt responsible for what happened to him.

Occasionally in the middle of the night Terry would whisper my name and from years of this happening I'd already learned that he was going to tell me he had to go number two. In that case I'd have to get out of bed; get myself awake by turning on the bedroom, hallway, and bathroom lights and make sure the toilet seat was down. Next I'd go back into the bedroom, pick him up and carry him into the bathroom while pulling down his pyjama bottoms and put him on the toilet. I'd then go back into the bedroom and give him a few minutes of privacy. After he told me he was finished, I'd go back into the bathroom: and pick him up, wipe him, pull up his pyjamas and carry him back into the bedroom and put him in bed again. I'd always make sure he had the old bleach bottle that he used for a pee-bottle (urinal) between his legs in case he had to urinate during the night.

Then I'd go back into the bathroom: flush the toilet, wash my hands, and go back to bed and try going back to sleep. I said try to go back to sleep because by this time I was wide-awake from having to concentrate on doing what I had to do so much. My ability to go back to sleep after doing something like that lived next door to being impossible to do when I'd already been to sleep once already.

Other times he thought he had to do a big-job and I'd go through the entire procedure of putting him on the pot, and go back into the bedroom to wait for him to say he was finished and then he'd say he didn't have to go after all. He called this 'having a pou-attack' and it used to drive me crazy because I was always left wide-awake when it was over with. Then I'd have to spend the next couple of hours listening to the purr of him sleeping until I fell asleep. Usually at night though, Terry would fall asleep fairly quickly because I'd hear his breathing purring like a kitten after a few minutes. Other times his breathing would be loud and bothersome. To make him stop making so much noise, I learned all I had to do was say his name out loud a few times to disturb his sleep pattern and he'd be quieter. Sometimes there was no sound coming from his bed at all and I'd get so spooked that something happened to him that I forced myself to pick the scab off that bit of curiosity and I say his name out loud until I got some sort of reaction from him. Other times during the night Terry would start crying and because I didn't understand what was happening I would ignore the sobs I was hearing. I've beaten myself up so badly over the years for this that it's amazing I've never had to pick up my teeth with broken fingers.

Chapter 9
In His Past

I first met Heather in September 1969 when the students from Mary Hill Junior High School (present day Pitt River Middle School) started going to PoCo and I grew to like her so much that I wanted to do something for her now that we were in grade twelve. I didn't know exactly what I wanted to do; I just knew I wanted to do something.

When I found out she had the lead role in the musical *Hello Dolly*, which PoCo was going to stage in May 1971, I saw my chance. I was too late to audition for a role in it and asked the director if I could be his assistant. He said yes. When rehearsals started in January 1971 I worked my tail off by going to two rehearsals a week and doing all kinds of other things for the play in between. When the play started its run I became part of the stage crew (changing the sets between scenes.)

PoCo High couldn't get it together enough in 1970 to put out an 'Annual,' so in May I joined the 1971 Annual Club to do my part to ensure an annual came out in my last year of school. My job was to write all the grad comments and because I didn't know everything about everyone in the graduating class and because time was running out I let it be known to the grads that they were to submit what they'd like to see written about them in it to Mr. Yip, who would give the information back to me to paraphrase. A lot of people did what I wanted them to do, but over sixty-five people didn't. The people who didn't do what I asked them to do and I both share the responsibility for the blank space under their pictures equally.

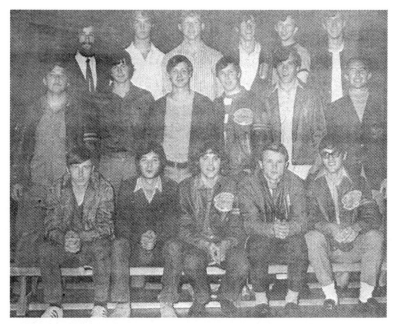

1970-71 PoCo Senior rugby team front row centre.

TP (short for Terrance Patrick), as Terry told me he wanted to be nickered at this time, must have phoned PoCo and found out when my rugby team's home games were being played, because almost every home game we played I'd see Mom and him parking the station wagon on Sefton Street, which runs parallel to the playing fields at the back of PoCo.

They were never there to hear our team try to scare the cleats off our opposing team when we were giving a blood-curdling Highland Charge as we kicked off because Mom had to drive from where she worked in Port Moody to Vancouver to pick TP up and then she had to drive back to PoCo again. By the time she got back to PoCo the game had already started. The field we played our home games on was so polluted that I've still got scars on my legs from the infections I got from playing there.

It was never said directly to me, but I started to understand Terry was sicker than I thought he was. I figured that out when I saw he was getting weaker and weaker and asking me to empty his pee-bottle with less and less urine in it because he was having trouble lifting the bottle.

Attending PoCo's Awards Day Ceremonies at the end of the school year was one of the highlights of the year for me. I'd never won anything at any of these ceremonies before because I'd never done anything extracurricular around the school to deserve to win anything. I always went anyway because I liked seeing who won what. I knew that 1971 would be the last year I'd be able to attend a ceremony so I made sure I went.

I ended up winning a Major Service Award for doing what I thought was fun, a Major Drama Award for trying to impress Heather and a copy of the school letter (a big P, for PoCo, nickered the Big Block) that a few other rugby players were presented with at that time. When I was walking home with the two pins I'd won in my pocket and twirling my copy of the school letter around my finger I started thinking I had the world by the ear and nothing bad would ever happen to me.

Nobody was home when I got there, so I didn't show anyone what I'd won when they did because I didn't think I'd done anything special to win those awards. Besides that, I didn't want to divert any light off of TP because he'd been transferred to a different hospital because he was starting to get really sick at that time.

Jackie started going out with this big Italian guy named Alfredo, who put me in awe of him the first time I met him because when I was showing off how strong I thought I was by lifting some barbells over my head with two hands with a lot of weight on them, he simply lifted them over his head with one hand like they were made out of balsa wood.

Mom helped me buy a white 1963 Austin 1100 that she'd found for sale in Port Moody for $500.00 and Dad helped me get an afternoon wiper job at the Coquitlam Rail Yards Roundhouse (where Shaughnessy Station Mall is today) The wiper job was an easy job to do: turning engines around on the turntable, refuelling them, cleaning the engine cabs (where the crew sat), and making sure there were little cans of purified drinking water in ice buckets on the engines. My last two weeks of working there were spent cleaning and repainting shelves at the CP Rail's supply depot that was a few hundred yards north of the Roundhouse. The work I had to do there was so easy I should have felt embarrassed getting paid for it.

I didn't want to believe the chest infections that TP was getting were as serious as they were until August 10, 1971, when the entire family was told to go to Vancouver's Pearson Hospital (where TP had been transferred to because he was really sick.) Our neighbour, Walter Borke, picked Dad up at work and drove him to the hospital. When Mom and I had gotten to TP's room, the first thing I noticed was that he was inside an oxygen tent to help him breathe easier. Mom was going to feed him his favourite meal of fish and chips that my Aunty Wava's son, Jim, had brought for him to eat. He told her he wanted his big brother to feed him. So I got into the oxygen tent with him and started feeding him. He kept asking me if I wanted any, so I had a few chips. He kept looking over his shoulder and not saying anything, making me curious about what he was looking at. But I never asked him. After a while he started motioning behind him and asking me, "Who's back there?" I told him, "There's only a wall." But he kept looking behind him anyway.

When he said he was full I left the room by telling everyone, 'I need some fresh air.' I didn't want to say the real reason was because the situation had finally sunk in and the emotions in me felt thicker than paint. When I knew I was out of everybody's sight, those emotions started Niagara Falling out of my eyes so hard that I couldn't stop crying for fifteen minutes.

When I eventually went back into TP's room, the nurse (whose hard job it must have psychologically been—like most nurse's jobs are) came in the room and told us we should go because TP was starting to get too tired. We all said, "We'll see you later" to TP, and he said, "Good-bye" to everyone except Jackie, who he told, "Everything is going to be all right, and we'll have tea tomorrow." Jackie felt that he knew she wouldn't have left the hospital if he had just said good-bye to her.

For a few years before that, TP and Jackie would have tea together in the rumpus room almost every Saturday night and talk about the things that mattered. I was never asked to attend any of these teas because I wasn't the type of person to sit around and talk about important things.

My denial system told me that nothing bad was going to happen to TP but he must have known he was going home (dying) because he wanted me to feed him his last meal.

Mom and Dad and I drove home with the car radio turned off and barely a word spoken. TP was still so big in my mind that I went over to Mr. and Mrs. Borke's house with Mom and Dad, so I wouldn't be alone.

After a couple of hours I walked back home and tried to cry because I knew a person felt better after a good cry and the sigh that follows. But I couldn't cry any more because my tear ducts were empty and I started doing the things I thought TP would like to be doing instead of being in that hospital. I watched TV and I listened to two of his favourite rock & roll groups, Creedence Clearwater Revival and the Beatles, for a while, and went to bed for a restless sleep.

At 3:10 in the morning on August 11, 1971, TP took his final breath and Mom picked up the ringing telephone beside her bed when the hospital phoned to tell her what had happened. There was a short beat of silence and I heard Mom crying the cry of a mother who would never see her youngest child alive again. TP only had seventeen years in his past.

Chapter 10
Feeling It Too Much

Mom and Dad drove into Pearson Hospital to positively identify TP's lifeless body, and to answer whether they'd allow experiments to be performed on him or not. Mom and Dad told the doctors that the family wanted an open-casket funeral and that they could do anything they wanted to him, but they had to leave his eyes and hands alone. I should have gone upstairs and joined them when they returned from the hospital, as a sign of family unity, but didn't. I just stayed in my room like an ostrich, hiding from the reality of the situation instead.

Shortly after that I realized the last thing TP had said to me was 'Good-bye.' So I installed an inner reminder in myself never to say good-bye to anyone to this day because I'm afraid it might be.

I knew I was one of the main characters chosen to play a major role in the real-life movie of TP's life, and I knew I'd never be able to make it up to him for all the time we never shared together.

The summer I graduated from high school turned out to be the last time I ever cried like a baby. The crying had nothing to do with leaving PoCo's hallowed halls behind me, or being grateful I'd finished school's twelve-year prison sentence, or missing the feast of friends I'd made over the years. It had everything to do with everything surrounding TP's graduation from life and how sorry I felt for myself that I hadn't treated him better when he was alive.

Mom and Dad donated TP's wheelchair to Sunny Hill Hospital. And I thought everyone I knew would know about his passing, so I didn't phone and tell anyone about it because I was all messed up. The following month when I was talking to Susan on the phone and told her what happened to TP I found myself being asked why I hadn't told her about it when it was happening because she would have wanted to share my grief with me.

I put myself through a lot of mental anguish over the next few months where I felt I'd stolen TP's last bit of recognition from the people I hadn't told about his passing.

I'd already decided to follow through with my plans to attend Douglas College (which was being held in trailers at Eighth and McBride in New Westminster at that time) in September 1971 because I wanted to take something to do with English because I liked fooling around with words so much. When I started going to classes at Douglas the first major difference between going to high school and going to college I noticed was that students were allowed to smoke right in the classrooms at college at that time. I thought that going to college would be as easy as going to high school was for me, so I never talked to a counsellor at the college or anything and ended up taking five heavy-duty courses in one semester.

Some of the members of the rugby team that I'd graduated with were going back to PoCo to play another year of high school rugby so they could go to Europe and play there. I didn't want to go back to high school just to play rugby.

As it turned out Douglas College had a rugby team so I decided to play one last season of it before I ran out of youth. I was under the impression that a lot of my new team mates on that team were more interested in partying at the Cariboo Hotel than they were into playing rugby. I was used to playing on a championship rugby team in high school but felt a lot of the members on the Douglas team didn't care what the outcome of the games they played were. I was upset at this because I could have gone back to PoCo and played on that team, and gone to Europe and played there.

Many of the other players on the Douglas team were doing a lot of drinking, but I knew I was still a lousy drinker and always got drunk fast and didn't like losing control of what I was doing. I still wanted to fit in with them and usually drifted away from them after a while when the temptation to start drinking the way I wanted to drink started counting itself down to drink the way I wanted. As the invisible peer pressure began working on me more and more, I started drinking more and more with all the quirks that go with what my mind-set was telling me a wild and crazy rugby player was supposed to be like.

Suddenly I got upset about the way my life was going and began acting the way I thought I was supposed to act more and more. It wasn't long before I was drinking before I went to these practices and home games to get that artificial courage a wild and crazy rugby player like me wanted. When rugby season ended for the semester I found myself so broke that I couldn't pay attention to anything and just stopped going to college. I didn't officially withdraw or anything. Instead, I went into Vancouver and applied for a job as a switchman at CP Rail because Mom had once told me that the CP Rail likes to keep railroading in the family.

I'd gone into Vancouver to apply for the job that morning and before I even got home that afternoon CP Rail had phoned Mom and Dad's house and told Mom I was to report to the CP doctor in Vancouver for a physical in a couple of days. I passed my physical and began my training and six-month probation period with two other guys in late November 1971. We spent a couple of days learning the fundamentals of the job by working a few day shifts in the Coquitlam Rail Yards. One of my first nighttime shifts I did was done at the Vancouver Rail Yards that started around midnight and it was the first snowfall of the year. I had never driven a car in that much falling snow before and had to drive from Port Coquitlam to Vancouver in it. I wouldn't let a simple thing like falling snow stop me from doing what I wanted to do because I'd already proven to myself that I could do anything I set my mind to do because I played rugby for all those years.

That first shift that I did in the Vancouver Yards was done at a railroad crossing after going through the tunnel that the Skytrain would eventually use. When I was coming home the next morning I was given my first traffic ticket. It was from a Vancouver cop for driving down a one-way street the wrong way, and for not having the snow wiped off my rear window. The cop followed me for a block with his lights flashing silently for attention behind me and I still didn't see him. The only reason I noticed him at all was because he hit his siren for a heartbeat.

One day when it was snowing fairly hard I told Dad I'd give him a ride to work. After dropping him off at the Roundhouse where he was to get the engine he was running that day, I drove around the Roundhouse's parking lot and came back a few wrist shakes later and climbed on his engine, telling him I was working the Second Westminster Branch with him—which goes into New Westminster. We'd seen each other quite a few times at work before, but had never worked together before. I think Dad was proud and nervous that day; proud he was working with his own son, and nervous I might get hurt working in all the snow on the ground. Dad was as sensitive to things at that time as I am sensitive to things today, and because the principle of 'like father like son' is as true today as it's ever been there is no use talking about Dad's character because they are still in me today.

That was the one and only time we ever worked together.

In February 1972 Mom co-signed a loan for me and I bought a brand-new 1972 Toyota Celica. After I had the car for a while I met some people from high school and we did a bunch of drinking together and I got snookered. One guy had a motorcycle, and because I was filled with the brave new world of youth that told me that nothing bad would ever happen to me, I drove that motorcycle all over the Mary Hill area of Port Coquitlam for the fun of it. I didn't wipe out or anything, even though I didn't know a motorcyclist is supposed to lean with the bike when turning corners.

I took a girlfriend to her high school grad and had a few bottles of beer before the after-grad party we were going to and passed out in my car in the driveway of the party house for a few hours while she went to the party house alone. When I woke up a few hours later I didn't know where I was, but luckily for me my homing instincts were still turned on and I followed them home.

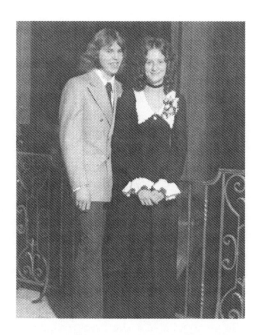

May 1972.

When my six-month probation period on CP Rail was about to end, I found that I wasn't getting as much work as I was expecting to get. I started to get some scaredy-cats about not having enough money for my car payment that month, so Jackie helped me get a job in construction with Alfredo's brother in North Vancouver for the day. The night before I was to work for Cory, Mom told me to drive the Celica over to Alfredo and Cory's house and get a ride to the job-site with him. I agreed to do that. But by the time June 16, 1972, yawned itself awake, I decided not to take her suggestion because I had convinced myself that bad things would bounce off me.

It was a 'fry an egg on the sidewalk' day at work that day and when it ended I went against my own better judgment to the bar with a bunch of the other workers for a few beers before going home. I had thought about not going for the blink of an eye but decided to go anyway because it was the first time I could drink with a bunch of older guys. It was the first time I felt accepted as a man by other men. I felt great. After drinking two or three quick glasses of beer I started feeling the effects of what I drank and left the bar before I started feeling it too much.

My Second Life

Chapter 11
Living It

I drove a few blocks from the bar and had a head-on collision with a bus at the corner of Fourth and Queensbury. An ambulance picked me up and took me to the emergency room at Lions Gate Hospital. The hospital staff did what they had been trained to do by finding out who I was and told whoever answered the phone what happened.

Shirley was over at Mom and Dad's house helping Mom wash the evidence of heavy smoking off the kitchen ceiling before going to the Commercial for a few glasses of beer when the phone started screaming for attention. Mom reacted to it in her usual way by picking it up and saying 'hello.' She listened for a beat of time (turning white with extreme seriousness) as Shirley saw something bad had happened.

Mom was told that I'd been in a serious car accident and it was strongly suggested to her that she and Dad get to Lions Gate Hospital as soon as possible because it didn't look like I'd be surviving that much longer.

Shirley's head was screwed on better than what Mom's was, and she took charge of the situation by making all the arrangements to get Dad off his engine and meet them at the Coquitlam Yard Office so she could drive them to the hospital.

Ten months before this, Dad was called off his engine because Terry was so sick. It rarely happened that an engineer was ever called off his locomotive, but twice in one year was almost unthinkable.

The Friday night bottleneck traffic in the little town of Port Moody that they had to drive through to get to North Vancouver was so congested with traffic that they thought of having the Port Moody police escort them to Burnaby where the Royal Canadian Mounted Police would guide them the rest of the way to North Vancouver. But Dad said in an anxious, frightened manner, "If we're meant to get there on time, we're meant to get there on time, and there is nothing we can do about it." So with a few gallons of wishful thinking, crammed down the throat of anticipation, that they'd make it to the hospital in time to see me alive, they plugged ahead.

The blood had been washed off me by the time they arrived at the ER and seeing how Shirley was only a family friend and not a relative, she wasn't allowed to see me and was told to wait in the waiting room. She wondered what greeted Mom and Dad.

When the three of them saw each other later, Mom and Dad supplied her with the answers to that puzzling question her imagination was asking itself. My neck was swollen out to the width of my head and it looked broken to them.

At the time Mom and Dad were seeing me, Shirley had been busy phoning Jackie at her apartment in New Westminster and telling her about what happened to me. Jackie headed for the hospital right that very second. It hadn't even been the first anniversary of Terry's passing yet, and she might be losing her other brother. Going from the eldest of three to being an only child in the family in ten months is hard to imagine, isn't it? No wonder Jackie doesn't want to think about those times today!

Meanwhile Mom was ranting and raving about how she was going to sue the tires off BC Hydro (the name of the bus system in the lower mainland at that time) for causing the accident, but a friendly nurse told her about the beer smell in the air when I was brought in and Mom was quiet.

Shirley always felt the accident wasn't totally my fault, but because I reeked of beer when I got to the ER the bus driver was found innocent of any wrongdoing and the blame was firmly placed on me.

For the next week Mom and Shirley went to the crash scene over and over to try and figure out what had happened to cause the accident. They concluded that at that intersection most of the bus drivers flicked on their turn signals to say they wanted to pull into the bus stop on the other side of the intersection before they even entered it. This would imply to drivers like me, who were not used to seeing buses all the time, that the bus was planning on turning the corner instead of going through the intersection to the bus stop on the other side.

I lay in the Intensive Care Unit struggling to stay alive, with my body taken off manual and put on cruise-control, where my body automatically does everything it has to do by itself, and hooked up to various tubes while my family and friends visited and talked to me every day to keep my brain stuffed with as many thoughts as possible, because it had been discovered that if an unconscious person's thinking is forced to operate, that person has a better chance of survival. Even a radio playing in the same room is enough to stimulate an unconscious person's brain.

As time passed my family started worrying if I'd stay in that vegetative state forever, and were secretly asking themselves, would I end up being crippled up and be hampered by a wheelchair, a walker, crutches or a cane forever?

Skip and his mom saw me so often at Lions Gate that they thought their car could find its own way there. Most of the people I'd spent years going to school with stopped thinking about everyone else they'd gone to school with soon after graduation and were too busy getting into their own futures to think about me. I can't blame them for that because the most important part of life is living it.

PoCo man injured in crash

A 19-year old Port Coquitlam man is listed in serious condition at Lions Gate Hospital today following a collision with a B.C. Hydro bus in North Vancouver Friday.

Gerry Phillip Williamson of 1792 Jensen in Port Coquitlam, was the lone occupant of a car that collided with the bus at Fourth St. and Queensbury at 5:30 p.m.

North Vancouver RCMP reported that the bus driver and passengers were not injured.

An investigation will be conducted.

Newspaper clipping reporting my accident.

Chapter 12
Improve Physically

Doctors and nurses were always in the ICU on a twenty-four-hour-a-day basis making sure the unconscious patients were okay. The turning point for me came fifty-two days after the accident when the calendar read August 1972 (nearly two months). Mom and Dad were visiting me that day, hoping for some kind of a change in my condition because I was moving around more than usual.

Some ICU nurses were talking about going for their coffee break near the bed I was in when I said 'coffee' like I was part of the conversation and slipped back into my coma.

Hollywood depicts a person in a coma suddenly waking up and talking like nothing had ever happened more than a good night's sleep, but reality debunks that theory.

When they heard me say that one single word everyone got excited because I was now out of the living-dead state of existence further than anyone at the hospital had seen me before. It would have been unrealistic to expect a full recovery at this stage; in fact I'll always be recovering because I'll never be like I was before the accident again. I started believing everything in life revolved around me at this time.

I received what is called a Traumatic Brain Injury in the accident. A concussion is like a bruised brain, and the term 'head injury' stretches its meaning from hurts such as scalp wounds and bumps on the head to canyons dug into the skull. But the term TBI is the actual disruption of the normal structure and function of the brain where the brain cells themselves received some disturbance and didn't get enough oxygen for normal function. A head injury is more or less temporary, where a brain injury is permanent, meaning forever.

When I had regained consciousness my body stopped running on cruise control, and was put on manual again. As I became more aware of my surroundings the hospital staff was forced to restrain or tie me to the bed so I wouldn't get out of it and try walking around on my own. Being tied to that bed frustrated me because my mind told me there was nothing wrong with me but the restraints were telling me there was.

The physiotherapists started working on me as soon as I moved from one state of existence to another because nobody wanted my body to atrophy more than it already had, and I was transferred from the ICU to a ward called the activation unit, where I started getting physically active again.

It had been so long since I'd done anything physical with my body that the subconscious thinking that goes into doing anything physical wasn't there anymore. My thinking was so confused and messed up at that time because nothing seemed to work the way it used to.

When it started looking like I was going to survive, Mom and Dad made plans to take over power of attorney of my financial affairs because they didn't know how much I'd come back to being normal due to the amount of brain damage I got and no one thought I'd improve that much at that time. The first prognosis by the doctors is always bad because if the patient doesn't improve to the point the doctor said they would, the doctor would be considered correct, and if there was improvements past the point the doctor said the patient would get, the doctor would also be correct—a win-win situation.

If I said I remembered everything that happened in my life at this time, I'd know I was lying, and because I don't want to lie to you I'm going to have to rely on what other people have said happened and filter those memories through mine. To the best of my ability I'm going to truth you.

Being out of the coma wasn't the first or the last phase of my recovery; the emphasis had only shifted from concerns about my survival to improving the quality of my life. One of the first bits of rehabilitation I did was done in what was called 'mat class'—where I sat on a mat on the floor and did such exercises as lifting my feet a short distance off the floor for the count of ten, and slowly lowering them. This was hard on me at first because my brain was telling me I could still do fifty sit-ups and push-ups without breaking into a sweat while reality was proving I was having a hard time even lifting my feet off the floor. In other words, my memory didn't forget what I could do at one time, but I couldn't do what I wanted done.

I was put in a wheelchair, but I worked hard to get out of it because wheelchairs reminded me of Terry so much. This in turn brought back the memory that I hadn't appreciated him as much as I should have when he was alive.

I didn't forget everything I knew before the accident—I just couldn't remember some of the most important things as clearly as I once was able to. I don't know how long it took before these memories came back, but they did come back. The things I used to be able to do without thinking about were now the hardest things for me to do because they required constant thinking and rethinking about doing before I tried doing them. Not being able to do these things made me explode into fits of anger, causing me to speak my mind when I should have been watching my words.

My first memory after I regained consciousness is of throwing a glass of water on an OT who wanted me to do occupational therapy when I was trying to sleep a headache away that I was constantly having for the first few years after the accident.

I was now in the unique world of someone with a head full of memories that they used to be able to do things a certain way and were now finding they couldn't do what their thinking said they could.

As my awareness about myself grew I realized that something serious had happened to me, but I wasn't sure what that was. The past, present and future were shrunk into here and now. The next few months were confusing to me as I was discovering just how helpless I really was.

During that time I tried doing some of the things I could easily do before the accident by doing hours and hours of monotonous physiotherapy. I now had a different style of walking called a gait that I didn't have before my accident. I started thinking my life was a serious cross that I had to carry around with me all the time and I believed this new life I was living was a life sentence and that I'd be living forever.

At a meeting with a Lions Gate doctor, he explained what happened to me by telling me that my brain was scrambled. I couldn't understand what he was saying at that time, but I didn't forget it either. The times my family came to visit me were the most important times to me because they were people I felt connected to. My mind told me they were going to be at Lions Gate at the same time every day, so as far as I was concerned they had to be there at that same time every day or my thoughts would start doing flip-flops in my mind. Expectations of their arrival got so bad that I sat in my wheelchair so close to the elevator doors that other people wanting to visit their friends had a hard time getting off the elevator.

Over the next few years Mom and Dad and Jackie were constantly reminding themselves of this fact. I don't mind that they did that today because I wasn't aware I was doing it at that time. And by the time I realized it, it was so far in the past that it didn't make any difference to me anymore. In fact, I like it that they remember it today, because it ensures this little mental snapshot of a memory will be remembered in the future.

I didn't like talking to people I didn't know very well at this time because my speech was so slowed that it embarrassed me. As a result, I thought everyone would think I was a freak, or worse—by treating me like one if they heard me talk. I began to notice that I wasn't remembering the things I wanted to remember all the time at this time. It seemed I was always distracting myself into doing something else besides what I intended on doing.

I decided I wanted to smoke cigarettes again after not smoking for a long time because I smelled cigarette smoke in the air. Mom and Dad told me to ask my doctor first. I believed they thought I'd forget I ever smoked at that time, but my will to smoke was stronger than my willingness not to smoke and I started going through the dizzy spells that I had gone through when I first started smoking.

Mom and Dad were giving me five small packs of cigarettes every week to smoke, and when my smoking increased, it increased past the point I'd ever smoked before. Consequently I always ran out of smokes before the week ran out of days, because it seemed that I was trying to make up for the lost time I was forced not to smoke.

When I ran out of my own smokes I started bugging the other patients and their friends on the activation unit for some of theirs. After a while I was told not to bug everyone for smokes. I still wanted to smoke, so an orderly said he'd give me some if I cleaned bedpans for him.

Word that I was smoking more than usual must have got back to Mom and Dad because they started giving my smokes to the nurses to dole out to me. I was asking them for so many that the nurses started telling me they were too busy to stop what they were doing to get one for me and asked me to ask them later. I'd usually forget to ask for one for a few hours. This controlled my smoking.

I spent hours and hours, days and days, for weeks and months doing physiotherapy during the week and not doing anything to help myself improve on the weekends because I've always believed that weekends were a time to take it easy. And because everything was being done for me by everyone else, I wasn't doing anything to make myself get better. I eventually realized I wasn't improving as fast as I should be, and it was going to take me longer to get better. As soon as I understood that I got out of my wheelchair and forced myself to push it around empty to break the hold those feelings held over my head. I pushed that wheelchair around empty because the act of pushing it would convince me I wasn't in it, while the activity of pushing it made me improve physically.

Chapter 13
The Happy Hooker

I was well enough to go home for the first time. That was one of the greatest feelings I've had in this new life of mine because it showed me I was getting better. Mom and Dad both came to Lions Gate to pick me up that Friday night. They put me in the back of the station wagon, the same way Terry rode in the car, because I didn't have enough strength to hold myself up, either. And they didn't know what else to do with me. Feeling that made me determined to stop flopping around some day, but I was powerless over it at that time.

We stopped at my Aunty Wava's apartment in Burnaby long enough for my cousin, Rick, a member of the RCMP who would die of a heart attack chasing a bad guy on August 31, 1983, to come out to the car and talk to me for a while before starting on our way again.

The scaredy-cats I was feeling from going home for the first time made me feel carsick, causing me to ask Mom to pull the car over to the side of the road every so often to wait for them to pass. Those feelings of nausea eased as we got closer and closer to home while the thrill of going there made me start giggling. I managed to hold the giggling in check after a while.

Part of the reason I wanted to curb my laughing was the anticipated surprise party I thought would be happening for me when we got there. But when we pulled into the driveway it became obvious there wasn't going to be any party for me because no one was waiting for us to arrive. I realized that I wasn't as popular as I thought I was at this time.

I was so upset about this that I retreated into myself and forced any memory of the first time home out of my mind.

Every week the orderly on the activation unit would sit me on a bath chair in the shower room and spray me with water like he was washing his car. I hated having to take showers like that. It bothered me so much that I made up my mind that I would start giving myself my own shower as soon as I could.

My uncle Frank, who was a wounded North African tank veteran, was always telling me that the only place I could find sympathy around him was between shit and syphilis in the dictionary whenever I wanted everyone to start feeling sorry for me, because he had to go through the same experience in the 1940s that I was going through in the 1970s.

One night I had a vision that told me I wasn't going to end up being crippled, gimped and gibbled for the rest of my life if I started doing what I was being asked to do in physiotherapy more vigorously. I started doing the exercises the way I was being told to do them more aggressively, and I stopped believing the fallacy that was trying to convince me that just because I'd once been a fancy-dancy rugby player I wouldn't have to work on myself as hard as others had to. I started to believe that my past had passed and there was nothing I could do about it.

Like anyone else who had been hurt in a serious accident, I too hoped I'd go to bed one night and wake up the next morning to find I'd only had a bad dream about being hurt. I had to teach myself to stop thinking like I was or I wasn't ever going to improve.

In the past I'd always thrown myself headlong into any situation to think about quitting without a fight, but the answer to this dilemma was staring me in the face, but I couldn't see the solution to this problem because I was too busy looking for the hardest answers to the simplest questions. I decided to go with the flow to see how it went. I felt the fear and did it anyway.

I suddenly understood that I was only feeling sorry for myself, and was waiting for the day I'd get better without putting any effort to get that way—I was waiting for something to change me without putting in any of the effort to make that change. By taking it easier on myself

I started along the road to a happier future. I realized this new adventure didn't work the way I thought it should, and I realized I had to get so sick of how I was feeling about the way my life was going that I was willing to do anything to make that change. The easier things became the simpler my life became and I started working on my ability to walk more. As time moved to the back of the bus, my walking got better and better.

If I hadn't changed my way of thinking about how my life was going I'd still be waiting for my life to change today. All the hoping and praying in the world wouldn't do a thing to change me until I put the effort it took into changing myself.

My new job in life was to start doing everything the way I did when I wanted to keep playing on that championship rugby team in high school. I've never forgotten what I learned about myself on that team, and when I applied that knowledge to this new life I was starting to live it helped me want to change what I didn't like being anymore. If I kept doing what I was doing before that group of thoughts sank in, I'd still be getting what I was getting at that time, zilch, zip and nada.

When that decision sank in, I started doing everything the hard way. I did absolutely anything to make my life tougher. After doing everything that way for a long time I found my life was getting easier and easier and I started to wonder why I found it so hard to improve in the first place. When I put down that cross I was forcing myself to carry I started to improve. By simply accepting myself as I was, I soon started getting better.

After I was released from Lions Gate in late 1973 I was allowed to take a shower by myself for the first time. The feelings I got from giving myself that first shower meant so much to me because I knew I was doing everything that needed being done. Even if it was only a quick shower it was long enough for me to know I could do it all.

Sure, Mom might have been standing outside the bathroom door (ready to rush in and help me if I fell down) but that didn't matter because I knew I was doing it all.

I was still sleeping upstairs in Mom and Dad's room at that time, but after giving myself that first shower I felt independent enough to sleep in my old bedroom downstairs again, and started putting pressure on Mom and Dad to let me sleep in my bedroom again. Eventually I was allowed to.

Now that I wasn't in Lions Gate anymore everyone in my family saw there was something different about me. As the clocks started moving faster and faster with the cadence of reality it became obvious that something was seriously wrong with me. When these situations became too obvious to overlook anymore, Mom and Dad got in touch with the community health office in Port Coquitlam for some kind of help to cope with me.

The Health Department in Port Coquitlam at that time (future Mental Health) must have gotten brain damage confused with mental illness because I was put into the same category as people having mental problems. My brain was so messed up at that time that I thought I was well.

When BC Hydro started running their buses out to Port Coquitlam from Vancouver in 1974, Mom and Dad tried convincing me that I could take the bus to all my appointments in downtown Port Coquitlam by myself. But I balked at this for a long time because I thought I was too messed up to take the bus anywhere alone. Over time I started thinking I was supposed to take the bus as if it was some kind of punishment for being in the accident. The first long bus ride I took by myself was to see Heather at her apartment in the Gastown area of Vancouver. We went out for dinner and drinks and I got so wasted that I had to be driven home.

Another time when Heather and I had illegally parked her car on Granville Street and went somewhere to do some shopping, and had returned to the car, a Vancouver police officer was writing a ticket for the car. He recognised me from when he and I had played on the same Douglas College rugby team and ripped up the ticket.

I met an attractive red-headed girl, who was a cast member of *Hello Dolly* in high school, riding on the # 980 bus one day and got Brenda's phone number from her. But my brain forgot I had her number and I never phoned her. In fact, my memory about everything was so bad at this time that I was afraid it would never improve. But the speed of my memory's recovery improved at the same rate as I improved physically.

In order to help me get my act together mentally, I was told I'd have to go to Burnaby Day Hospital on the corner of Willington and Canada Way as an outpatient, in February 1974. I didn't want to go there at first, but it turned out to be a nicely run place where we'd be given a nice hot and healthy lunch and two coffee breaks every day. I had to take three different buses to get there in the morning, and after a while I found that taking the bus wasn't that bad.

I told myself that I didn't have the same kind of mental problems that a lot of the other people at Burnaby Day Hospital had, and that it was only my TBI that was making me different than everyone else. I decided to make myself feel better about the way I was by having Gordy (the guy in charge of the PE department there) instruct me enough to earn a junior swimming badge.

For the next six weeks I would be at the indoor swimming pool at 8:00 am for my swimming lesson until I was a good enough swimmer to earn the badge. I did one more sit-up and push-up than the day before to get warmed up, and then I'd swim lengths of the pool and other things to earn it. When I was being tested for the badge, I showed off to my nurse, Carol, and my OT, Maggie, my ability to earn the badge because I was as proud of myself as if I was a little kid again because now I knew I could get better.

After people had been clients at Burnaby Day Hospital for a while, they'd get to show a newer person the way things were supposed to go around there. When my turn came it was with a Vancouver girl who had a recreational drug problem (a junkie) that was making her hair fall out. She was still a pretty girl and because of that I'd do absolutely anything she asked me to do. One Friday she wanted to leave early and I said she could because I wanted to people-please her. Monday morning that girl and I were the stars of a special meeting between staff members at Burnaby Day Hospital who told me that she had done drugs the night I said it was okay for her to leave early and I wasn't supposed to show her the ropes anymore because I was not dependable enough. Everybody has done a few things in their past that they wish they had never done, and I guess I just told you one of mine.

After finishing with Burnaby Day Hospital, Jackie came up with the idea that I should start hooking rugs to improve my eye/hand co-ordination because it was so bad at the time and all I was doing with my life at that time was a lot of nothing. So she bought me a rug-hooking kit and I became the happy hooker.

Chapter 14
The Way I Was Before

A woman who room-and-boarded with one of Mom's friends was driving home from work one night and was hit by a train in the fog. Karen was in a coma, not as long as I was, but she suffered a TBI as the result of her accident. This doesn't mean she wasn't hurt as bad as I was, and in case you're wondering, brain damage doesn't depend on loss of consciousness at all. Everyone thought Karen's injury and mine were the same because as far as everyone was concerned all brain injuries are the same. But every brain injury is different. We were all hurt in a different way so it stands to reason that our brains were affected differently.

By far the worst problem I was having at that time, and still bothers me today, is my ability to remember things. Another big problem I still have today is losing my balance. When I first became aware I was always losing it I tried to control it, and was always losing the battle and getting mad and frustrated because I kept falling down. So in essence, losing my balance controlled me the same way a slow driver controls the drivers behind them by making them mad and frustrated.

I learned to control falling down at home by planning the routes I'd take when walking anywhere in the house—by having places like walls I'd use as touch-points all the time.

A survivor of a TBI can experience any of the following combinations of symptoms or none at all:

Expessing everything in a wordy roundabout way
Dfficulty following through or finishing things
Difficulty in remembering the right word to use
Difficlty speaking smoothly, easily and clearly
Problems with getting along with other people
Needing supervision in almost everything
Difficulty in thinking clearly and effiently
Misunderstanding what is said by others
Incresed use of alcohol or illigal drugs
Repeating things over and over again
Difficulty planning and organizing
Difficulty in setting realistic goals
Difficulty in following directions
Difficulty in dealing with change
Problems with co-ordination
Decline in social activities
Lack of interest in things
High or low sexual drive
Changes in personality
Dependency on others
Doing things slowly
Problems with taste
Changes in appetite
Sensitivity to noise
Poor concentration
Sleep disturbances
Loss of confidence
Hearing difficulties
Temper outbursts
Easily distractible
Dizziness/vertigo
Lack of stamina
Visual problems

Being forgetful
Mood swings
Hallucinations
Mood swings
Restlessness
Poor balance
Easily bored
Depression
Impatience
Loneliness
Irritability
Anxiety

Karen walked from her place on Coquitlam Avenue the five or six blocks over to Mom and Dad's place every Monday, Wednesday and Friday and the two of us would spend hours and hours playing Cribbage, drinking coffee, smoking cigarettes and talking about whatever was on our minds. This was more therapeutic for us than we knew at that time—proving that the blind can lead the blind.

Skip and I had gone to the Golden Ears beer parlour (since torn down near Shaughnessy and McAllister at that time) for a few glasses of beer every once in a while, and I discovered I could go there whenever I wanted to. The first time I went in there by myself a big tough tattoo-laden guy told me to leave. So I walked out of the bar and stood on the sidewalk and thought he had no right to tell me I wasn't allowed in there and went right back in. The guy was still sitting in the same spot and started laughing when he saw me, and I knew it was okay to be in there.

That first time was quite an adventure for me because I discovered beer was only two bits a glass and for two or three bucks I could get pretty well gooned and forget about the way I was for a while. I had no argument with getting as drunk as I was getting because I didn't realize that brain-damaged people were affected so relentlessly by alcohol at that time, and believed I was just a cheap drunk.

A guy I knew from high school told me not to let my drinking get out of hand. As the years were sliding into the past Skip and his girlfriend,

Bet, were always telling me not to drink as much because I was always breaking out into these ugly drunks whenever I drank. People in my family were constantly telling me I shouldn't drink so much because it would slow my recovery down, but I ignored all of them.

It seemed I was always getting drunk, so Jackie tried to make me want to control my drinking by telling me I was probably allergic to beer, and that I should quit for a week to see how I felt. I didn't drink for almost a week, and by the end of those seven days I was feeling so good that I was almost dislocating my shoulder patting myself on the back that I rewarded myself by starting to drink again because I proved to myself that I could control my drinking. I found out years later that if you have to control something it means it's already out of control.

One day I met quite a few guys at the Ears who remembered me from when we played rugby on the same team in high school, or they reminded me I knew them. It didn't take very long to learn to accept the free beer these guys seemed to be buying me whenever they saw me in there, and as soon as I started to accept it, the feelings changed from accepting it to expecting it.

These rugby guys were buying me beer all the time and after a while I started thinking it was neat that I could go into the Ears with a dollar in my pocket and be given glasses and glasses of beer and not have to pay for them. I'd stay until these rugby guys all went home and pick up all the loose change left on the table as the waiter's tip and have some more beer. The waiters must have told them about me taking all the change and drinking the dredges (leftover beer at the bottom of glasses) because eventually they stopped going to the Ears to drink. They simply disappeared, leaving me with a bunch of rugby players I didn't know.

As time staggered away I became nothing more than a 'cling-on' (a person who clings on to other people and treats them like they are their only friend). After getting known by the newer members of the rugby club for a while, I was taken to their clubhouse for a party they were having. I stayed there for a few hours, drinking their beer until I felt I didn't belong there anymore and got up and left, thinking I was ending my relationship with rugby forever because I realized I wasn't the way I was before.

Chapter 15
Without a Hitch

Skip invited me to Prince George to see him and Bet. They were living there because his employer had transferred him there. To get to Prince George I took a twelve-hour bus trip, and when the bus pulled into Cache Creek for a leg-stretching break, some guy riding the bus with me told me there was a bar at the hotel that we could go to and have a glass of beer and make it back to the bus before it left. I had a gut feeling I shouldn't trust this guy but I ignored it. I went in the bar with him and settled back for a few glasses of beer. What I didn't know at that time was that brain-damaged people don't know how fast or slow time passes and when the guy left the table (I thought he was going to the bathroom when he was actually leaving for the bus) I just sat there.

When I became aware that this guy had verbally sucker punched me (twenty minutes later) I went outside and found the bus had gone. I was told that another bus was due to leave from there in a couple of hours. I knew I had to catch that bus because everything I had for the trip was on the other bus. When the other bus picked up passengers there in another few hours I thought of the proper words to say to the new driver so he'd let me take his bus into Prince George. When I eventually got to Prince George I spent the day playing miniature golf with Bet until Skip got home from work.

There was a fair at Prince George that weekend (like Port Coquitlam's May Day) that we went to. I met my cousin, Jim, who was working for the carnivals at that time (that's where Skip and Jim first met and eventually found out they had both been Queen Scouts.) Time has erased the rest of the weekend from my memory, but Skip reminded me years later that when it was time to go home on Monday morning, this different bus driver wasn't going to let me take his bus because he thought I was too drunk and would bother the other people.

Skip got ticked off at this and did what a good friend is expected to do, and explained what had happened to me before the driver would let me on his bus. Incidents like that had been happening to me for so long that I had stopped thinking they were any big deal. That's when I started thinking I was being treated like my intelligence had sprung a leak, but I knew that there was nothing wrong with my intelligence, and that it was just being misdirected.

I always thought that people believed I was slightly retarded, bone-headed, feeble-minded, or just plain stupid when they treated me like that. But, they were actually treating me like a drunk when I was sober. Strangers who don't know me still treat me that way when I'm physically tired, or I'm play-acting today because I do such a convincing job of it that people don't think I'm acting at all.

People get scared when they don't understand something, don't they?

I wasn't doing anything with my life besides becoming a 'no-mind,' when my family decided I should clean lumber (taking nails and other construction paraphernalia out of wood) at Jackie's boyfriend's job site in Haney, as Maple Ridge was called then.

I'd only earn a hundred dollars a month working there because that's all I was allowed to earn each month on disability insurance. It wasn't much of an incentive as you can tell, but earning that hundred bucks a month was better than not earning anything at all, and was teaching me how to work again and giving me self-esteem.

Alfredo would pick me up at 7:30 each morning during the week and take me to where he worked. As soon as we got there he'd start putting out extension cords and connecting them to the skill saws that the other carpenters used during the day. At first I just stood by the truck waiting to begin work, but after a while I started feeling guilty that I wasn't doing anything and started helping Alfredo put out the extension cords. When I heard a whistle blown at 8:00 a.m. I'd go to where there were piles of wood with nails in them and take them out until the first coffee break of the day.

It was hard work for the first couple of months because I hadn't done anything physical for such a long time. But once I got calluses on my hands and it felt like I was wearing gloves, the work got easier. We'd work five days a week and a half day on Saturday because, as Alfredo once told me, "You have to work hard when you're young so you can take it easier when you get older."

I didn't like working on Saturdays because it meant I had to go to bed so early on Fridays. Since I was trying to make up for the time I stayed home on weekends in my teenage years I believed Fridays were a night to stay up and party on. After that job was finished we worked at another site and another one after that.

After a while I started feeling independent and began taking the bus to these new job sites. I'd always get the address of the new places we were going to be working at on Monday morning on the Sunday night before we were going to work at these new places. This meant I'd have to figure out how to get there by bus for 8:00 the next morning. At first I used to phone bus information to find out how to get to these new places, but eventually figured out that the people providing bus information only gave me a route to get to where I wanted to go, but if I asked the bus drivers how to get somewhere they'd give me the easiest and most direct route to get to where I wanted to go.

I'm glad I learned that then because it taught me how to get to different places by bus easier. By learning how to take the bus I was given the freedom of being able to get to where I wanted to go without having to depend on other people for rides all the time. And believe me, that is a great freedom to have.

I was starting to drink beer pretty hard and was meeting exotic dancers at the Ears quite often. One day I was sent to clean some lumber at a Vancouver job site on my own, but went to see a dancer friend of mine when she was working in the skid-row part of Vancouver before I went to the job in the afternoon.

When I got to the construction site's address a few hours later, I cleaned a bunch of lumber at the wrong address before realizing I was supposed to be across the street cleaning lumber.

I started feeling sorry for myself because I had to work in all kinds of weather and talked myself into quitting that job the first chance I got. One day I was standing in the mud (with a hole in my boot) at a construction site near Coquitlam Centre when the time to quit that work slammed through my brainpan. After lunch I just walked off the job and went home. That was the first time I obeyed a gut feeling of mine.

One morning shortly after that I woke up with a sharp pain below and to the right of my belly button that Mom and Dad thought was only a severe case of hunger pains. I wanted to believe them because I'd been told I was wrong about so many other things after my accident that I thought I must be wrong about this too.

I ate the huge breakfast they prepared for me but the sharp feeling didn't go away. Question marks started dancing with each other in the back of Mom and Dad's minds about what to do about this pain. I remember Dad made a joke about it probably being a bone I'd swallowed in my sleep the night before and it had gotten hooked up on something in my stomach and hadn't finished digesting yet. They told me I should lie down for a while, so I did.

But the gut ache only got worse and I was taken to Leigh Square to have a doctor check me out. Three different doctors came in the examining room and gently poked and prodded my belly and brain with a litany of questions resulting in me going to RCH for emergency appendix surgery. The hospital staff at RCH had to wait a few hours to let my digestive juices have a good work out on my breakfast before they could do any surgery. If you don't consider the mark the incision left on my belly as anything to be concerned about, then everything in the operation went without a hitch.

Chapter 16
For That

On November 9, 1974, Jackie and Alfredo got married in a huge wedding ceremony on Alfredo's birthday, "so he'd never forget our anniversary," I remember Jackie saying at that time for some reason. Jackie wanted me to be a part of the wedding party so I became an usher. The rehearsals and wedding went without incident, followed by a fantastic Italian wedding reception at a rented hall in Vancouver.

Uncle Buck acted as emcee for the event. 'Bucky Roarky,' as he was nickered that night, started his emcee duties off by saying, "I'm Jackie's godfather," causing a bucket of laughter to be poured over our heads from the room full of Italians! The amount of food they served the guests was out of sight and out of mind. I had never been to such an elaborate event like that before.

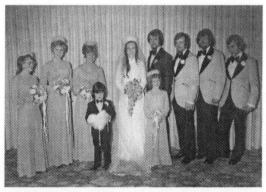

Jackie and Alfredo's wedding party in 1974. I'm on the right.

Time melted into early July 1975 and I was told I'd have to go to GF Strong in Vancouver on the 29th of the month to improve my balance and co-ordination. I didn't want to go to this place at first because I thought I was doing okay. But because it looked like I was limping on two legs when I was walking I had to go. I didn't feel I belonged there because I thought I was better off than a lot of the other patients there. After time had passed though, and I accepted the way I was I found the other people going there weren't as bad off as I thought they were.

My physiotherapist had me running on a little track that was there because I was into playing sports so much before I was hurt. I only tried running a few times before I stopped running because running felt so strange to me in this new life I was living. I ended my running career by saying, "I'll never try running again."

My teeth were bothering me a lot because I hadn't been to a dentist in years because I raised so much hassle at the dentist offices I went to. In August 1975 arrangements were made for me to see a dentist in Vancouver. He did hundreds of dollars' worth of work on my teeth that I don't think he ever got totally reimbursed for. My teeth were in such bad shape at the time that I don't think I have one single tooth in my entire head that doesn't have a filling in it. Dr. Fast and his trusted assistant, Vicky, got my teeth in good shape again.

While trying to make me want to change myself, my physiotherapist worked on my balance quite a bit. One of the things he thought would help me the most was to sit on a chair and play volleyball with other people in their wheelchairs or sitting on chairs. There were two classes of volleyball each day, the first and last classes of the day. When the initial idea that I was being forced to do this style of therapy had worn off, I started having fun doing it. The fun I was having became contagious and most of the people playing or watching the games got infected with enjoying themselves as well. The fun I was having became the high point of my day and because of that, it became the high point of the day for people watching the game as well.

At that time GF Strong had a pub night every second Saturday night and from that point onwards I was either drinking or thinking about drinking because my alcoholism was now turned on with an obsession. After I'd successfully proven to the staff at Strong that I was a drunk tearing through their lives, word must have got back to my GF Strong doctor who told me I wasn't allowed to go to pub nights anymore because I raised too much stink with the hospital staff when I was drunk.

A quadriplegic (someone who can't use their arms, hands or feet very well because of some neurological reason) who watched the afternoon volleyball sessions on a daily basis would take me out to his van to have a few cans of American beer every day during the week because I wasn't allowed to drink at pub nights anymore. We drank American beer because there was a beer strike going on at that time.

He drank his through a straw because it was easier for him. Other times when we didn't have anything to drink we'd spread some liquid hash on a cigarette and smoke it to escape the reality of being messed up like we were. And like in my teenage years, whenever I drugged I was still getting as paranoid as ever.

I've always heard and always believed that drinking American beer was like drinking apple juice compared to drinking Canadian beer and drank it that way because I believed what I heard. The American beer I was drinking at this time was drunk to escape reality but I didn't know it at that time.

I started taking the bus home on the weekends because no one in my family was offering to drive into Vancouver to pick me up. After taking the bus back and forth a few times I was surprised that no one was as excited about me being at home as I was, which contributed to me feeling unpopular there.

I was temporarily confused when some of my family members started talking about how I'd probably enjoy living in a boarding house when I got out of Strong. This was due to my constant inappropriate behaviour. But the more they tried getting me excited about moving into a boarding house the deafer I became.

I had learned that I could get back and forth between my house in Port Coquitlam and the skid-row bars in Vancouver that some of the other patients at Strong went to on the weekends quite easily when I was still going to Strong, and started going to these bars again because of the cheap thrill that drinking in these bars offered me.

When I started going back to these skid-row bars after I was discharged from Strong, the other Strong patients that were going there then started treating me like I wasn't with them because I was too much of a drunk. This made me mad at them because not very long ago they would have known I was like them because I was physically messed up too.

Jackie had a boy at the end of September 1975 that I was excited about because I hoped Jackie and Alfredo would name him after me. But they named him Mark instead of Gerry.

By the time I'd progressed from doing physiotherapy five days a week as an inpatient to doing it two days a week as an outpatient in October 1975, beer drinking had become one of my best friends. I eventually understood that if I wanted to get any better physically I'd have to do the rest myself. But because I was so sick of doing therapy around this time I decided to take a holiday from it for a few months.

After not doing anything with my life for a while I asked if I could go back to PoCo to see if I really was a slow thinker, like the way strangers treated me. I also wanted to make myself feel like how I felt when I was a student at PoCo in 1971. Arrangements were made for me to take English 12 again in January 1976. When I started attending classes there my English 12 teacher turned out to be a former grade-twelve student at PoCo when I was a grade-eight student there.

A few days after starting school again, I met a guy I'd known since we were kids. It took me by surprise seeing Doug so grown-up because in my mind he was still a little kid, and here he was so much older. I hadn't realized he'd gotten older while I was getting better.

Doug was always with a good friend of his. This reminded me of Skip and me when we were in grade twelve because we were best friends too.

As the year progressed and I was in the school's hallway I saw this friend of Doug's rubbing his right knee or thigh because it had fallen asleep or something. I didn't think much of it at the time, but I never forgot it either. The only reason I remember him at all was because he had the same first name as my brother. He was Terry Fox.

I passed English 12 and the only girl I met was named Rhea, who came to my house a few times, because I lived so close to the school. I eventually gave her a book of my favourite song lyrics and poems for her birthday.

In October 1976 I read a letter from a lady named Sharon telling me I might benefit from a place in Port Coquitlam called 'New View Society' because the after-affects of the accident made it appear I was mentally handicapped.

I was excited about being able to go there until someone in my family put the idea in the back of my mind that the place was for ex-mental patients. Since I had never been in a mental institute these family members didn't think the place applied to me and I refused to go there because I was being told that I was wrong about so many other things since my accident that I thought I must be wrong about wanting to go there too.

When you are being told that you are wrong about things for so long, you eventually start believing you are wrong about what you think.

I stayed at home quite a bit, and by staying home and not doing anything, I wasn't getting any better physically. When that piece of fruit ripened with the hands of time, I decided I had nothing to lose and went to New View one day to see what would blossom from going there. The redheaded director of New View (at that time) welcomed me to that rat-infested Dalkey Building (since been torn down but was beside the underpass at that time) when I first got there from the Ears. Because most people don't know that coffee only makes someone who was drunk a wide-awake drunk, I was offered a cup of coffee to sober me up. Coffee was only a dime there where it usually cost two bits in a cafe, and it was somewhere for me to go without having to spend a lot of money.

All it would cost me to get to downtown Port Coquitlam by bus from Mom and Dad's house was twenty-five cents if I went there when it wasn't rush hour or thirty-five cents in rush hour. In those days rush hour went from when the buses started running until 9:00 a.m.—not rush hour all day like it is today. I made sure I didn't leave the house before 9:00 a.m. each day so I could save the additional dime.

One day I got to the Ears before it was open and because I didn't want everyone driving by the hotel seeing me standing there waiting for the bar to be opened, I walked to the back alley to wait for the doors to be unlocked. When I got back there, there were at least three or five or seven other people doing what I was doing.

I finally got power of attorney over my finances back again and seeing how I thought I had an inexhaustible supply of money, I bought quite a few rounds of beer for strangers because I had convinced myself that if I bought beer for them they would want to be my friend. But I was wrong about that, because all they really wanted from me was the beer I was buying them. I decided to buy something for myself before I ran out of money and bought a stereo. I paid cash for it and had them deliver it to Mom and Dad's house. When it got there I discovered I didn't have a clue how to put it together and phoned my cousin and asked him to put it together for me for a case of beer.

I started feeling sorry for myself again because I realized my life hadn't turned out the way I'd planned for it to go and started taking the bus into Vancouver to drink in the skid-row bars to try and get the same feelings I got when I was at Strong again. But drinking there at that time didn't feel the same way anymore. I remember one time I felt swanky for some reason and started drinking beer in the swankier part of Vancouver and being asked to leave the bar because I was too drunk and finding myself back in the skid-row part of Vancouver again because I felt comfortable drinking there. I even got cut off there for being too drunk and falling down and knocking people's beer over.

Another time I went for a drink in the skid-row part of Vancouver because it was only a little ways down the street from where the bus stop was at Hastings and Main (nickered Wasting and Pain—where nothing dies of old age) and decided I didn't want to drink there anymore because this guy offered to knock my teeth down my throat unless I bought him a beer. An angel, disguised as a waiter, overheard what was being said and told the guy to get out of the bar. This not only saved my teeth going down my throat, but also made me think there were probably lots of angels disguised as people walking around.

When I was bombed and riding on the bus going back to Port Coquitlam I'd always bother the other passengers riding on it too. I remember a couple of times the bus driver inviting me to get off the bus because I bugged too many people too many times.

If I was tired when I got on the bus I'd go to the back of the bus and lie down on the rear seat and have a nap. If there were people sitting there when I wanted to be lying there, I'd simply toot a few loud and nasty smelling beer farts and breathe beer breath on them until they got too uncomfortable or nervous that I'd fall or get sick on them and they'd give me their seats.

My cousin, Jim, who had become a bus driver by this time, picked me up a few times at various places in Vancouver when I didn't know what I was doing. He pretended he didn't know me if I was too drunk. I can't blame him for that.

Chapter 17
To Do with Myself

Somehow that few months I'd given myself to party it up in after leaving Strong ended sooner than I expected and I found myself doing more and more drinking in Vancouver because I developed a powerful drinking habit and didn't want the people in Port Coquitlam seeing me drunk all the time.

I went to my cousin's wedding reception in Seattle, Washington, and when I got bored with what was happening there I decided I wanted to have a beer in a tavern because I had never been in a tavern in the US before. I left the reception and walked onto the street and asked the first people I met where a tavern was. They told me to walk a few blocks up a street they pointed to and I'd find one. So I walked uphill (towards skid-row) dressed to the nines looking for a tavern. It wasn't long before I found one and started drinking in it.

I quickly discovered that the American draft beer I was drinking in this tavern wasn't like drinking apple juice at all because I was getting as blitzed, swacked and drunk as ever. When I ran out of American money I left the tavern to go back to the reception because no one in the tavern would lend me any money. When I walked onto the street I found I didn't have a clue where I was. All I knew about where the reception was that it was downhill from the tavern because I remembered I had to walk uphill to get there. I walked all over the place trying to spot a landmark I recognized before the searching party of relatives found me.

Jackie and Alfredo had another son at the end of January 1977 that I was excited about because I was sure my first name would be part of the baby's name this time. But Terry's name was used in Steven's name instead, which was just as good.

I had been smelling things that no one else seemed to be smelling ever since I had my accident and decided not to tell anyone because I was afraid they'd start calling me a dog if I did, because dogs smell things before people smelled them. Skip's mom had always told me she noticed me smelling my fingers and said I should try to break that habit if I could.

I didn't know at that time that having a heightened sense of smell is a characteristic that many brain-damaged people share.

When I was still in high school and doing sit-ups on the hardwood floor in the gym I'd always get a slight pain at the end of my tailbone that lasted for a few minutes after I'd finished doing them. At that time I never thought much about it because those sore feelings always went away soon after they started. But increasingly in 1977 that pain started bugging me worse than a fly buzzing around my head that I couldn't chase away.

When I got home following a slouching session after a long bus journey, I would have to spend the next half hour massaging that whole area because it was irritating me so much. One day I discovered there was a sore seeping some kind of bodily fluid that didn't smell very good. I told Mom about this and she made an appointment for me to see the doctor at Leigh Square because she didn't want an encore of my appendix problem. I showed the doctor what my problem was, and was put in RCH to have a cyst removed in a couple of days. The surgery turned out okay and I was out of the hospital a few days later with the suggestion not to do anything too vigorous for a few weeks.

The day I got out of the hospital was a Friday, so of course, I had to go to the Ears to see my drinking buddies—the same ones who were too busy doing nothing to visit me in the hospital when I was in there. A new dance floor had been installed at the Ears when I was in the hospital and I decided to dance on it because I loved to dance at that time. Besides, I thought the warning I'd been given didn't apply to me because I suffered terribly from a generous case of terminal uniqueness and believed things didn't apply to me unless they were specifically said to. Like, I thought drinking and driving were illegal only when you were caught doing it so I had done a lot of drinking and driving. I believed it didn't apply to me because I'd never been caught drinking and driving before.

I must have had a good time that night because the next morning I felt terrible and could barely talk. When Mom asked me about how my operation was doing I showed her what was going on with it. She took me to Leigh Square as soon as possible because it was in pretty bad shape. After I was examined by the doctor arrangements were made to put me in St. Mary's Hospital in New Westminster (that has since been torn down) to let my wound settle down a bit. But being in that private room I was put into caused my brain to start thinking I was put into solitary confinement and I decided I wanted to leave the hospital. The hospital staff must have phoned home and Dad came to get me. He must have been terrifically upset with me because the tension in the car was so thick that I had to open the window to breathe. After I got home and was resting in my room Mom and Dad must have phoned Go, who was now living in Port Hardy on Vancouver Island, and asked him to come over to the mainland and take me back to his place for a few months to get me away from the bad influences in Port Coquitlam.

Go came over and picked me up and we took the ferry, using the Inside Passage, that took us directly to Port Hardy because driving his truck all the way along Vancouver Island to Port Hardy would have been too bumpy for me. When we got to his house his wife, Tina, took me to the hospital to have me checked out. The doctor there decided to keep me as a patient for a week to have special baths of Epsom salts and water for an hour, five times a day to let my wound settle down. The hospital in Port Hardy at that time was on portable trailers while the new one was being built. Between baths I would wander around that single-floored hospital and talk to the other patients to stop myself from going bonkers while stuck in there.

One day when I was wandering around the hospital like a head with its chicken cut off, I met these guys who gave me a beer 'because you look like you need one.' (Drinkers sometimes like to help other drinkers.) It turned out that their buddies were leaving all kinds of booze outside their window for them to have a drink whenever they wanted. And seeing how it was Port Hardy, where it rained freezing rain or snowed every single day I was there, they always had access to nice cold beer.

When I was released from the hospital and had returned to Go and Tina's house I continued taking those baths four times a day now for the next month. At first I just sat in the tub for that time, but after the boredom got to me and before I started going wacky, I bought the fattest book I could find, and started reading it for the time I was sitting in the bathtub. After a month of taking these baths my wound was healed enough where I didn't have to keep taking them. I then found myself in Port Hardy with nothing to do, so I started going to a bar to see the dancers during the day, and every night I'd go for a few glasses of beer after dinner.

When I had gotten back to Port Coquitlam I was so broke that I started going to New View for something to do. A few months later a student working there for the summer, named Anne, told me her favourite performer was Van Morrison, where one of mine was Jim Morrison. I wondered if the two performers were related in some way. When I look at the picture of Van on the inside of the *Moondance* CD, and compare it to the cover picture of Jim on *The Doors* CD, I ask myself the same question.

Anne also told me she and some friends were organizing the first Vancouver Folk Music Festival, that was going to be held in Stanley Park on the second weekend in July in 1977. It felt like she was asking me to get involved in it, but my brain got folk music confused with cowboy music and because I've always been a true disciple of rock and roll (hating any music that wasn't) I never looked into what folk music was all about.

Skip asked me to be best man at his wedding in Coquitlam on New Year's Eve 1977. I also remember the date on the invitations said the wedding was going to take place on December 31ᵗʰ instead of December 31ˢᵗ by mistake for some reason. Being best man for my best friend's wedding was a once-in-a-lifetime experience that sticks out in my mind in Technicolor.

I was at New View one day in 1978 and met a guy who told me he was looking for a roommate. Because I didn't feel as popular at home as I once did, and had already concluded that I was old enough to live on my own, I told him I'd move in with him. After a month of living at this guy's trailer I decided I didn't like living there anymore because he had this little dog that peed on the floor all the time. It seemed I'd always be the one whose bare feet would find these cold puddles that the dog left on the floor.

At the same time, I was offered a job by one of Alfredo's brothers in Haney (picking up garbage a couple of days a week). I felt glad about being offered the job because I'd never done any work like that before.

Most of the time the work was fairly easy but there was the odd time I worked my buns off. Actually it was harder taking the bus there than doing the work itself. So I asked Mom to look for a place for me to live in Maple Ridge. She found a brand-new apartment on 119ᵗʰ Avenue for me to rent and I was moved in within two weeks. The apartment that Mom was shown wasn't the same one I ended up living in though. I ended up living in an apartment that was above the driveway leading into the underground parking lot that no one else wanted for that reason. I got used to hearing the constant coming and going of cars after a few months. It wouldn't be fair to say the apartment manager at this building was taking advantage of the way I appeared to him at the time, but...

One day the driver of the garbage truck I was working on thought I was telling him it was okay for him to leave the spot we were at when I was only wiping the sweat off my forehead. He drove away leaving me standing there in the middle of the road. As soon as he left, I started running down the street after him yelling for him to stop. He didn't stop for a few blocks.

When I decided I didn't want to work on the garbage trucks anymore I began existing on my disability pension again. After the thrill of staying home all the time had worn off, I'd walk the block to the Lougheed Highway and hitchhike until the bus got there and go to New View. I hitchhiked because I'd probably get a ride before the bus got there in order to save money.

One day in 1978, a new director by the name of Kay started working at New View, adding a lot of class to the place. Kay immediately showed the people attending there that she cared more about the people attending New View than the previous director did. She would always sidle up to me whenever I was drunk there and compliment me on how inappropriate I was. She'd always ask me questions that I didn't want to think or talk about by throwing little digs at me that worked on my subconscious mind, causing me to remember what she had said for years to come. I knew that the answers to all these questions were that I was feeling sorry for myself because I believed my life was ruined because of the car accident. But I didn't want to tell her that because I thought she'd make fun of me.

I still thought about what Uncle Frank had said to me at times, and I didn't want to tell her I was getting drunk and sobering up when I wasn't there all the time. That didn't mean I drank a lot though, it just meant I did a lot of drinking because I didn't know what else to do with myself.

Chapter 18
Had Fallen There

I remembered Heather and after I found her phone number, I started phoning her when I was drunk and trying to forget the way I was at that time. One day I phoned her in a state of being three sheets to the wind (very drunk) for the umpteenth time, and because she was tired of me phoning her all the time when I was so drunk, and because she wanted to help me, she asked if I wanted her to phone a Recovery program for me and take me to my first meeting. That statement hit me so hard it didn't bounce off because I never forgot it.

Ever since I had my accident, when the most important things were happening, I didn't understand they were, and didn't notice that what she was telling me was one of the most important things I could hear in life. I thanked her very much for her concern and told her I didn't need those people to help me quit drinking while pretending to ignore what she was really saying.

I recalled the time when my Uncle Buck told me that beer never hurt anyone after I accidentally saw him taking a beer out of the refrigerator early one morning at the Jensen house. Because I thought so highly of Uncle Buck I told Heather that I only drank beer so it was okay I was always getting drunk. Besides, I thought I was too young and too smart and too good-looking to be an alcoholic. Heather said "Okay" and that ended the conversation and I kept drinking the way that I drank, even though the solution to the biggest problem in my life had been planted in the back of my mind. That was another time I'd been warned about my drinking by someone.

Somebody at New View mentioned that there was possible work at a sheltered workshop (a workplace for people with special needs) in Port Moody, and if I was interested in working there I should check it out. I said I would because I was bored with doing nothing all day and not having any pocket money all the time. I was finding it is just as hard on a person to not have any commitments as it is was to have some. I didn't think this place was going to materialize at first, but a few months later Hygrade Industries started operating.

There was another guy working there that first day who had already been shown how to work the cut-off, or chop-saw. He cut the pieces of wood while I stacked them. He tried his hardest to make me ask him to slow down, but because I've always been a sticking-to-it type of guy, I kept up to him. The next day when I went to work I was told the other guy had quit because he wanted a better paying job than the $5.00 an hour he'd make at Hygrade. Due to the fact that I'd already proven to the boss that I was a hard worker I was shown how the saw worked and became the new woodcutter.

I felt proud of myself for being the only woodcutter at this place because a few years before that I was in Lions Gate fighting for my life. That was the one and only time I was ever the number one employee on the payroll at a place I worked at.

I'd take the bus back home to Maple Ridge after getting on the Pacific Stage Lines bus in Port Moody and get off it in front of the Haney Hotel, nickered 'The Zoo' (due to what went on inside in those days.) Because the bus let me off in front of the Zoo I thought I might as well go into the bar for a couple glasses of beer. After I'd drank a few glasses I'd walk the block home, make my lunch for the next day, have something to eat and go for a few more glasses of beer before going home at ten or eleven.

One time, when I was at the Zoo, a girl asked me to go with her to her room and make love to her in front of her boyfriend. I was already in the bag (very drunk) when she asked me this question, so I went with her and did what I was asked to do until her boyfriend rattled a heavy-sounding chain and told me to get dressed and get out of there. After bumming a smoke off him, I left.

Years later I found out that was what was called 'a free ride'—where a boyfriend/pimp has a new prostitute show them they will do whatever the 'John' wants them to do.

One day a few weeks later I went to Jackie and Alfredo's place for a little chitchat and coffee. And because Jackie is a 'normy' (an 'earth person') she didn't offer me anything for sustenance besides coffee and food. Since she's also married to an Italian who makes his own wine, there was a bottle of grappa (Italian moonshine) sitting on the kitchen table from after dinner drinking the night before. Every time she wasn't looking at what was happening at the table I'd be busy pouring some into my cup of coffee, and before I knew it, the bottle was empty and I was drunk.

Jackie bawled me out for drinking all that wine in a tone of voice I interpreted to mean she thought what I'd done was funny. But on the inner side of my belly button I knew she was being serious. That was another time someone said something about my drinking to me, but I was too busy pointing an accusing finger at everyone else, and blaming them for my lot in life, to notice there were three fingers pointing back at me.

Life happened that way until late November 1978 when my boss at work came up to me and said, "Your mother wants you at home."

I got a ride to Mom and Dad's house from a co-worker, and as soon as I opened the screen door to the house Mom was right there and said, "It's Dad." I knew from the way she said it that Dad was dead. I remember saying without thinking the F word and Mom telling me never to use that word in front of her again.

CP Rail had to pull Dad's engine back to North Bend to put him on the ambulance for the trip to the hospital in Hope. By the time the engine was pulled back it was too late for Dad and I became half an orphan.

When the Coquitlam Yard Office first heard about what had happened to Dad they tried phoning Mom to tell her the bad news, but her phone was continually busy. So they decided her phone was off the hook and phoned her friend, Shirley, and told her what had happened. Shirley went over to Mom and Dad's place and broke the news to Mom.

No one knew how I would react to what was happening so I was taken to a psychiatric nurse who was a friend of the family. When I was at his house, I asked him if I could write the eulogy for the memorial service they were going to be having for Dad instead of a funeral, and was told to go for it. I was so upset that the family wasn't going to have a funeral for Dad like they had for Terry that I couldn't get it together enough to write anything, but promised myself I'd write one for Mom if I outlived her.

A few days later Mom asked me to move back home with her. I asked Little Billy to help me move back home because I remembered his mom had worked with Mom and he said he would, but when he came to my place to help carry the boxes to his van to transport them to Mom's house, he found that I hadn't packed a thing because my brain forgot to remember to do that. After we moved everything to Mom's place I made the decision to slow my drinking down quite a bit. I hardly drank anything for the first couple of months and noticed that Mom seemed to have given up on her life ever getting better for her, probably because life was so different now that she was a widow. To me, it looked like she was trying to commit suicide by using one of the two methods the law seems to allow—by smoking or drinking herself to death.

I realized that Dad had been coughing harder and longer when he first woke up in the morning when I was still in my teens. In fact it turned out that Dad died after he'd stopped his engine by taking his foot off what is called the dead-man's brake (that the engineer always keeps his foot on—that automatically stops the engine in case something like this happens) because of one those coughing jags.

Shirley quit drinking at the start of 1979 because she felt she was spending too much time away from her family. This really impressed me because I knew how much she liked to drink. She'd been one of Mom's best drinking buddies, and now that Mom didn't have anyone to drink with the two of us would go to different neighbourhood pubs for a few beers almost every Saturday.

Mom started telling me that her big toe was hurting her quite often, and she must have realized she was getting older and thought that because she'd spent so much of her youth taken off herself raising us kids, she decided to do what she'd always wanted to do—drink—because she started drinking more than usual at this time.

Today I realize that she'd gone through years and years of mental turmoil with the way Terry was and him dying so young, then me having my accident being too much for her.

Mom had started going to the #133 Port Coquitlam Royal Canadian Legion because it was more accepted for single women to drink there alone when the #133 was still on Pitt River Road, before there was a fire there and it changed locations. Almost every night when she came home from the Legion she'd knock on my bedroom door where I'd be reading, if I weren't out getting blasted. She'd walk in my room and start telling me about how old she was getting and how she was always feeling like the odd one out when she was with her girl friends and their husbands. And the tears would start rolling down her cheeks.

I wasn't helping her any because I was too far into the same problem she was into to help her find the answer to hers. I was so messed up from drinking at that time that I didn't know there was a problem to try and get out of.

Whenever I heard her car pull into the gravel driveway I'd start preparing myself for what would usually happen next. I knew she was going to come into my room. I knew she'd start crying until she ran out of tears. I knew she'd end up going upstairs to bed, and I knew I'd end up being upset over the situation. I didn't know how to handle what was going on, and never thought of asking anyone else for help either. Being the sensitive guy I am (like most Cancers are), I started drinking more and more to give myself the impression I wasn't bothered by it.

In June 1979 there was a wine and cheese party at PoCo called 'PoCo Comes of Age' to mark the school's twentieth anniversary. I'd already spent most of that day getting lubricated with beer at the Ears (I called my shift) because I felt so bad about being messed up like I was. We got a glass beer mug with 'PoCo Comes of Age' imprinted on it when we paid our fees to attend. I don't remember a thing about the whole night because I spent more time concentrating on the wine than on the people who attended.

Shortly after that I was walking home after my shift at the Ears ended, and noticed someone was having a house party at a house on the corner of Laurier and Kennedy. Without thinking of my actions I decided to join the party because I thought everyone in my neighbourhood knew me and wouldn't mind me dropping in for a beer.

But what I didn't know was that everyone else had changed when I hadn't, and I simply walked into the house and up the stairs and got myself a beer from the refrigerator and sat on the couch with everyone else and started drinking it. The guy who lived there noticed I didn't belong there and yelled, "WHO THE HELL ARE YOU?" I was so surprised that he didn't know who I was that I blurted out, "I'm Gerry, and I noticed you were having a party and decided to stop and have a beer." The guy started to make movements to physically throw me out, but Skip's younger sister (Pam) was there and I didn't get beaten up. Pam doesn't remember any of this anymore. As a matter of fact I'm surprised I even remember it because even though I didn't use my brain for anything other than keeping my ears apart for so many years, I didn't forget it.

In 1977, Terry Fox had his right leg amputated because he had cancer in it, and three years later on April 12, 1980, when Terry became confident that he had the cancer beaten he started running across Canada (The Marathon of Hope) to raise money for cancer research.

On May 18, 1980, I was mowing the grass in the yard and heard an explosion that was so loud that I turned off the lawn mower and walked around the house looking for damage to it because I was positive a car had smashed into it. I later found out that it was the eruption of Mount St. Helens in Washington State. Uncle Buck, who lived in Peachland, BC, told me a lot of the volcano's ash had fallen there.

Chapter 19
Any More

When I'd come home late at night I'd be as dainty as a rhinoceros with a broken foot. This would either wake Mom up or make her feel better because I'd made it home alive—making her hair turn white as she called it. I remember an Uncle Sandy, who died falling down a flight of stairs because he was drunk, having white hair too. So white hair probably runs in my family's blood steam.

Jackie and Alfredo had another boy in February 1980 they named Paul. I felt a little upset at them because none of their three boys were named after me. My oldest nephew, Mark, and I do share the same middle name though, and if Jackie and Alfredo don't have any more kids like they said they weren't planning, this would make Steve the middle child of his family like I am in mine.

There is also a saying that tells me I have to show respect in order to earn respect. And I knew I fell short of showing any of that in my performance as a human being.

Mom never came right out and said I was kicked out of the house, she just said she'd help me move to the Commercial instead. I didn't have a refrigerator at this hotel so making lunches for work was impossible. I didn't care about that because I could keep my beer cold in the tank behind the toilet easily enough.

Beer parlours were closed on Sundays in BC in those days, but every night that the bar was open there would be yelling and screaming in the parking lot when the pub closed for the night. This would wake me up and cause me to stay awake for hours because I've always had a hard time falling asleep when I've been woken up. After living in a hotel for a few weeks the novelty of living there had worn off.

One day Jackie told me that her brother-in-law (Cory) had a two-bedroom apartment in Port Moody that was vacant, and if I could afford the $300 a month for rent, I could move in there. I said I'd take it sight unseen, because anywhere was better than living at a hotel. When I moved into that apartment I thought I was living in Heaven because it was such a fantastic place to live: a block and a half to the #119 Port Moody Legion, three blocks to the liquor store and Port Arms (present day Jake's Crossing), five blocks to work and a few more blocks to grocery shopping.

I don't know when I joined the #133 Port Coquitlam Legion; all I know is that I had a membership card that would let me in any Legion.

I finally phoned Brenda and asked her out on a date. The day of our big date together though, I had already spent a shift drinking and when she picked me up at my apartment we went to the #119 to have a few glasses of beer. I didn't know that I was one beer away from being totally bombed when I drank it, so that's what happened when I did. Brenda never saw my apartment and I'm sorry to say this, but that was our one and only date together.

I wasn't sure if the #119 would let me transfer there or not but I applied to transfer there when my Legion fees for the next year were due. I knew that the #119's president had seen me drunker than drunk many times before at the #119, and he told me that they were going to have a board meeting in a couple of days and he'd let me know after the meeting if I could make the transfer or not.

Since there is no right way to do a wrong thing, and because I couldn't do anything to stop myself from getting drunk the day the #119's president was going to tell me if I could transfer there or not, I got absolutely sloshed because I figured I'd be allowed to join that branch because I'd spent so much time and money there. But I was told I couldn't transfer there. As soon as the president said I couldn't transfer to that branch I immediately became sober and went to Port Coquitlam and paid my dues for the coming year at the new #133 that was just west of the underpass and tried not to get as drunk in the #119 anymore.

Unknown to me, after Mom had done a lot of work around the yard at the Jensen house she started feeling pains in her chest and back, so she made a doctor's appointment and phoned Shirley to take her there. When the doctor examined her, Mom was told they were going to take her to RCH by ambulance because she was having a heart attack. She would have nothing to do with that, and said Shirley would take her there instead. Before she went there though, she had Shirley take her home to get her toothbrush and her own nightgown.

A couple of minutes after she was admitted to the hospital, bells and whistles began screaming and red lights began flashing— "CARDIAC ARREST, CARDIAC ARREST, CARDIAC ARREST." A temporary pacemaker was slipped into a vein in Mom's thigh and she was put into the ICU at RCH for a few days before she was stabilized enough to have a permanent one put in.

I think Mom started thinking about selling the house on Jensen at this time because she was probably feeling she was getting too old to take care of it by herself.

The only bad thing about living at the apartment on Mary Street in Port Moody was I was paying so much rent, which made it hard to entertain myself. It got so bad I contemplated quitting drinking for a couple of terrifying seconds before regaining my composure and cashing in my cases of empty beer bottles.

I was forced to say 'hi' to my old nemesis, Allan, when I was returning these bottles. I thought for sure I'd get a belt in the kisser this time too, but Allan just said 'hi' and was out of my life forever.

As I was walking one of the waitresses of the #119 Legion to her car after her shift ended, she stopped and said to me, "I saw you walk in the Legion not more than a half hour ago when you were sober, and now you look like you've been drinking all day." She paused for a beat of time to let what she was saying sink in, and said directly to my inner ear (so I couldn't help but hear exactly what she was saying), 'You are an alcoholic. That's exactly what you are, and you're going to stay that way until you get some kind of help."

Hearing a statement like that didn't make me want to stop, look and listen to what I was doing to myself, or anything. After walking her to her car I continued walking to the Port Arms beer parlour for a few more glasses of beer. That was another time someone had said something about my drinking to me, but this time I heard exactly what she'd said and filed it away in the back of my mind along with what everybody else had said about my drinking problem. Now I had a name for what my hassle in life was, and I didn't care any more.

Chapter 20
Ever Again

A couple of months later an extremely quiet guy working at Hygrade mentioned he was looking for a place to live. I knew we were complete opposites in every respect, but I mentioned I had a two-bedroom apartment with a vacant room in it to him anyway because I didn't think he'd be interested in being my roommate.

When he said he had to move out of his other place at the end of September 1980 I told him if he wanted to split everything right down the middle—rent, utilities, and food—he could move in. I fully expected him to say he wasn't interested in living with me, but he slapped me on the eardrums by asking when he could move in because the price was right. Later that same day he told me he didn't know how to cook and preferred I did it all. I said I'd do all the cooking if he did all the dishes, which he agreed to do, and we became roomies. Having Tom move into the apartment at the start of October 1980 gave me more money to spend on stuff I couldn't afford when I was living there alone. It meant I could drink more than before too. So I did.

Tom and I got along so well because we didn't do anything that bugged the other guy. Every morning my alarm clock would yell, scream, hoot and holler at me that it was time to get up. I'd have three or six cups of coffee before I felt awake enough to go to work. Tom on the other hand, would get up without using an alarm clock, have a glass of water and we'd head off to work.

On Sundays we'd walk to Save-on-Foods when it was in the Old Orchard Shopping Centre on St. John's Street in Port Moody, and pick out our food for the coming week. We'd bag it ourselves because that's what we did at that store in those days. It became obvious to me that I could eat better with two of us paying for the food rather than paying for it by myself. Usually I picked out what we'd eat because whenever I asked Tom if he'd like to eat something, he would always say yes to whatever it was.

In November 1980 my favourite rock star of all time (John Lennon of the Beatles) came out of the retirement that he'd been in for five years with the release of a bunch of singles that I went to different record stores in Vancouver and bought all in one day. I was glad I got them that day because on Monday, December 8, 1980, when I was watching TV and having a beer in the living room while Tom was in his room watching *Monday Night Football* with Howard Cosell, he came into the living room and told me that John Lennon was just shot outside his apartment in New York City.

I remember going to the Leon Hotel (where The Golden Spike is today) as soon as I could, to tell the disc jockey playing the music there what happened. But I made the mistake of having a glass of draught beer at the bar first and forgetting why I'd gone there in the first place. I still wonder what happened to that copy of *Double Fantasy* (the last record John and Yoko had released before John's assassination) that he had signed for his murderer earlier that day.

A few days later, during the ten minutes of silence his wife, Yoko, wanted everyone to spend in remembrance of John, I realized what I was doing to my life and decided to quit drinking as a sign of devotion to John's memory. But that abstinence only lasted a few hours. As more light shone on John's killing, I started thinking that John had predicted his own death in his song called 'Scared' from his 1974 album *Walls and Bridges*. It later came out that his murderer was jealous of John, and hated himself.

For another bit of trivia, on most of the Beatle record jackets the first two Beatles to die were beside one another (John and George.)

Tom moved out of the apartment at the start of April 1981 because the apartment was sold, and I was on another pub crawl (drinking in different bars) working my way to Jackie and Alfredo's place at the end of another two-week drinking binge when I met some former rugby players at one of the bars and we decided to have a few glasses of beer together because some rugby players are like that.

Time pulled me out of a black-out I was in the next day, when I was riding on a bus in a drunken stupor still thinking it was the night before, because my mind told me I was going to Jackie and Alfredo's place for a visit then. When I walked into their place at 11:30 that Saturday night, they were quietly watching television in their living room. My short-term memory's power of recall kicked itself back into remembering what I'd just done a few minutes before and it 'accidentally-on-purpose' jumped out of my mouth. As they were going up one side of me and down the other about my drinking, a thought flew in one ear and out the other telling me they'd forget all about what I'd done if I told Alfredo I'd done it for him.

From what they said though, I understood it meant they didn't want anything to do with me if I kept on doing what I was doing.

I'd just reached the basement of my life.

My Day of Reckoning had arrived.

Hearing them say that and adding, "And that goes for your mother too," I knew I'd better do something about my drinking or no one in my family would want anything to do with me ever again.

My Third Life

Chapter 21
But…

Life had suddenly gotten too real for me.

During the night a moment of clarity reminded me of what Heather said about that Recovery program years ago. I knew that I needed to change something in me and was willing to do whatever I had to do to do that.

Terry Fox, who was the Athlete of the Year when I went back to PoCo in 1976, died on June 28, 1981, from cancer, leaving us to finish the Marathon of Hope for him.

On July 2, 3 and 4, 1982, I was invited to an event called the Pacific Northwest Conference at the Royal Towers Hotel in New Westminster with these Recovery people. I didn't want to go at first, but was told there would be a free meal in it for me if I went. It was insinuated that I had to get rid a lot of my character defects before I could change myself more.

I found that by recognizing these characteristics and admitting to myself they were there and doing whatever it took to get rid of them they were slowly being removed. As time passed I noticed that people were being friendlier with me by inviting me to go out for coffee with them. This scared me at first, but I accepted it as part of my new way of life and I changed even more. The more I changed the more I wanted to keep changing because I liked these new feelings.

I started taking more showers and stopped swearing as much because I discovered those were two of the main reasons why people wanted to stay away from me because I understood that no one wants to be around abrasive people. I continued to drink until I heard someone tell my inner voice, "If you want your life to change, don't drink; because if you don't drink you won't get drunk, and if you're not getting drunk all the time your life will get better." I knew I had to change and now I knew what I had to do to make that change. I figured out that no one had ever been on my back about my drinking and were only on my mind about it. Karen, that TBI friend of Mom's, sublet her apartment on Coquitlam Avenue to me after Mom decided I couldn't live with her any longer. The apartment was only a block away from the Commercial so on November 25, 1981, after moving all my things into the apartment I told her that I'd buy her a few glasses of beer at the Commercial for helping me move. Mom and I went into the bar and Mom headed for the 'biffy,' as she called the bathroom, and I found a chair and sat down. A waiter, who had been serving Mom and me beer for years, put two glasses of draft beer on the table and left.

Because the habit of drinking was still so deeply imbedded in my personality I drank half of one without thinking of what I was doing and suddenly understood I needed more help quitting drinking than I thought I did. I understood that I wouldn't live long enough to make every mistake myself and decided to learn from these Recovery people's mistakes and do what these people suggested I do.

I just had my last drink of alcohol.

Because I knew that people don't come back to things that don't work, I decided to keep coming back to this Recovery program.

I lived in Karen's apartment for a year before Karen sold it and I started living with Mom again. During that time Mom started complaining about having a sore foot quite a bit. I never told her to have the doctor check it out because a child can never tell a parent to do anything. After all, they will always be the parent and you will always be the child.

I had surrendered my driver's license to an RCMP officer, who came right to the Jensen Avenue house to get it from me after I got out of Lions Gate. At first I thought it would be impossible to get my license back, but after a few inquiries were made I found it was possible to get it back.

Because I got my driver's license back I stopped thinking my life was a life sentence, and started believing it was an adventure!

When I got the actual license in the mail in another week, I found it had a bunch of restrictions on it that I wasn't expecting to see. These restrictions successfully restricted my ability to drive more than you could imagine.

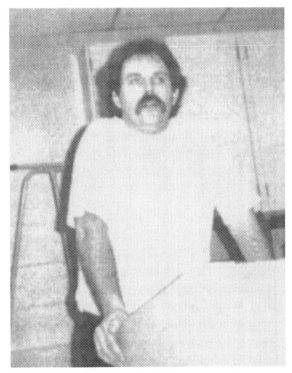

Me in 1983.

All I did for the next two years was concentrate on not drinking and not ruffling any feathers in anyone. This turned out to be a twenty-four/seven proposition for me because just doing the kinds of things that kept me away from starting to live my old way of life again, created a bigger change in me than I expected.

It made me want to do things I'd never wanted to do before.

Life was now about other people.

One of the things I did at that time was volunteer doing 'patterning' with a TBI girl. Patterning is retraining and stimulating the senses of the brain by repeating exercises over and over again to try and put them into use again. I also helped people with multiple sclerosis at Chimo Recreation Centre in Coquitlam.

I didn't want to change everything about myself at first, but I discovered that changing these bad habits were getting in my way to becoming a better person in this non-drinking life I was starting to live.

I'd always been a major heat-bag (someone who draws negative attention to themselves and inadvertently to the people they were with) and discovered I'd stumbled into another support group like New View Society without knowing it.

Not long after that I was over at Jackie and Alfredo's house having a coffee and was busy coughing up a storm after lighting up a cigarette, when eight-year-old Steve comes charging into the house. He politely waited for me to finish my coughing exercise and tossed a stinging message into my thinking, by saying, "Smoking is bad for you."

I heard what he was saying, and never forgot it.

He didn't know it at that time, but saying those few simple words caused me to look at my smoking harder than I'd ever looked at it before because I knew that what he was saying was the truth. I realized Steve was as smart as a sting from Lucifer, and it told me I'd better do something about my smoking before it did something to me the way it did something to Dad.

I knew I was smoking the way that Dad used to smoke because I always remember when I was a teenager Dad always had a smoke burning in an ashtray (even while eating dinner) and I was starting to do the same thing at my place when I ate. I had figured out a long time ago that smoking wasn't good for me and had accepted this nasty habit of mine was something I would never be able to stop doing because it was such a huge part of me. As long as I thought smoking wasn't bad for me, it would be impossible for me to quit smoking.

Alfredo, who is a fantastic carpenter, told Mom that he'd build a suite downstairs at the Jensen house for her, and she could rent the upstairs to somebody if she wanted. But Mom exercised her independence and sold the house and Dad's extensive tool collection to one of her so-called friends at the #133 Legion for next to nothing. She didn't consult with anyone in the family about the prices she was charging either. I often wonder if she had been coerced into selling the house so cheaply because she was like a lot of people in society who like to please strangers more than her own blood.

Today I realize that Mom was like a lot of other people in society who eventually start treating strangers like family and family like strangers once alcohol has gotten their thinking in a head-lock. She never went overboard doing that, but...

Chapter 22
A Lot

When Mom stopped using Lucifer on me the strap was put into a drawer and forgotten about. Eventually it was given to Jackie and used on Mark, Steve and Paul until they became bigger than I'll ever be. And most likely it will be handed off to whomever makes Jackie a grandmother first.

In January 1986, I was offered a season pass to go to Expo 86. Before that, I didn't know if I was going to see it or not. I went to it the first day (Friday, May 2, 1986) and saw Princess Diana and Prince Charles driving around in a fancy car waving to everyone with their windows rolled up, because it was raining. I remember thinking at the time that I was glad I wasn't them because I couldn't imagine being so over-protected that rain couldn't even get to me.

Mom was living in the McAllister Apartments in Port Coquitlam and had stopped complaining about her foot hurting her all the time, so I thought she had that problem taken care of. I could still tell she was having a hard time when she walked though, but marked that down to her age. I never asked her if she wanted to go to Expo because she gave me the impression that she wasn't interested in going. I ended up going to Expo more than fifty times before I realized it was the quality of my visits rather than the quantity that counted.

The last pavilion I saw at Expo 86 turned out to be the final show of the BC Pavilion, on Monday, October 13, 1986—the day Expo 86 closed its doors forever. Since it was the last day there was an RCMP in red serge wearing his Stetson hat standing at the entrance welcoming everybody as they entered the building. There was another officer inside the entrance wearing his dress uniform as well. The two officers stood in front of the screen that showed the movie that displayed the diversity of scenery in BC. We were told we were the last group of people to see the movie during Expo 86.

A few months after Expo ended, I started feeling these feelings that felt like something too big was trying to fit through my intestines after I'd eaten greasy foods. One day, I was over at Jackie and Alfredo's house having a cup of coffee and noticed there were slices of watermelon sitting on a plate on the table, and because I hadn't eaten watermelon in years I started eating them my usual way (seeds and all) when suddenly I started having one of those attacks that I'd always get when I ate something I shouldn't have. My sister-in-law, Barb (who shares the same birthday as me), said that the same thing had happened to her a few years ago and her doctor told her she was having a gallbladder attack. She added, "That's probably what's happening to you right now."

The next day I made an appointment to see my family doctor to have him confirm or deny that was what was wrong with me. He agreed with my suspicion and I was put in RCH to have my gallbladder taken out as soon as possible. I asked a nurse if I could have my gallstones after my operation for a souvenir, and she said I could.

When I was being wheeled away from my room to the operating room I started talking to God and turned the results of the operation over to Him because I didn't want to worry about what was happening anymore. The next thing I was aware of, I was being wheeled back to my room from the recovery room.

As we were going by the smoking section (a special place where smokers could smoke in those days) I started craving a cigarette worse than I'd ever craved one before because I smelled cigarette smoke in the air. I recognized a girl from having a smoke with her at some other time and asked her if I could borrow one (smokers like to help other smokers.) She gave me one and I asked the nurse wheeling the gurney I was on to stop and let me have the smoke. She stopped, and because I should have passed out or something when I smoked that smoke the nurse waited for something to happen to me. I had the smoke without the usual side effects that the nurse thought I'd be having.

Good to her word (like what nurses' words are) the nurse gave me my gallstones in a pill bottle when I was leaving the hospital. They looked like little rocks to me, so I bit into the largest one to see how hard they really were. It shattered because they are not as hard as rock as the name implies, showing me that TBI's can do stupid things as well as anyone else.

On December 31, 1986, I was going to a New Year's Eve dinner and dance at the Port Coquitlam Recreation Centre with a bunch of other Recovery people and decided to go to a convenience store near there to get a large pack of tailor-made cigarettes because it was a special night with lots of cigarettes left in ashtrays to burn out. I opened the pack by the garbage can just outside the door and took the foil off both sides of the package the way I usually do when I know I am going to do a lot of smoking later on. The reason I do that is to save myself from having to throw the foil into the ashtray later on.

As I started walking back to the dance, it started pouring rain outside. I hadn't seen it rain like that for a long time, so I stood under the awning of the store until the rain calmed down before venturing out in it. This sudden down-pouring of rain took my attention off of what I was doing long enough for me not to see the step going down from the sidewalk to the ground and I fell flat on my serenity pouch (my fat belly—the way it was at that tine) as the pack of smokes flew out of my hand and scattered on the wet ground. The majority of smokes were now useless to me, and instead of getting mad at what happened I simply went back in the store and bought another pack of smokes. I didn't like having to pay so much money for the first pack, and then paying as much for the second pack bringing the total for cigarettes up to more than I wanted to spend. For someone living on a fixed/limited income like I was, that was way too much money to be spending on something I didn't need.

All night long I kept thinking of quitting smoking on Cold Turkey Day because I was tired of waking up coughing and sputtering like Dad did every morning: I was sick of the glorious headaches I was getting all the time, tired of the little holes burnt in my clothes, sick of having stained fingers. I was sick and tired of smoking.

I was thinking of what Steve had said to me years ago. I was thinking of all the pros and cons of smoking that I faced every day I continued smoking. And there were more cons than pros when I'd finished looking at all the statistics. The desire not to smoke became larger than the desire to smoke. I got off the debating team to quit or not to quit smoking because I finally understood that smoking was going to kill me the way it contributed to killing Dad.

Cold Turkey Day was coming up sometime in the summer, and I made up my mind I was going to quit on that date because it seemed like the right thing to do at the time. I had figured out that the only thing keeping me smoking was the thought that told me I could never quit smoking. As long as I thought that way, quitting smoking would be impossible to do.

I was taken by surprise at the start of January when I heard that Cold Turkey Day was going to be on January 21, 1987. That date was coming up pretty quick and I didn't even know how I was going to quit smoking yet! I had to learn what I had to do to quit fast, or I wasn't going to quit when I wanted to.

I was watching a news program on TV shortly after that and part of the program had a segment on it about how to quit smoking. My ears perked up when I heard that, because by this time in my life I believed that when the student is ready, the teacher appears from out of nowhere. The people on the TV supplied me with the answer to that quandary by telling me to pick a date I wanted to quit on, and ten days before that date I was to tell myself that in another ten days I'm going to be a non-smoker. The following day, I was to tell myself that in nine days I'm going to be a non-smoker. I was to keep that up until the last few days of smoking when I was supposed to start making myself excited about quitting smoking. So that's what I did until I could say to myself, "Tomorrow I'm going to be a non-smoker."

137

On January 20, 1987, at quarter to midnight I put out my last smoke. When I woke up the next morning I didn't want a smoke the first thing in the morning the way I'd done for as long as I could remember. Before that I'd always thought that I needed that smoke when I first woke up to jump start me into the new day, and I believed that if I didn't have it I'd spend the rest of the day feeling there was something missing. I spent a lot of time thinking about having a smoke that first day, which I was told was normal for a few days, but I didn't act on that feeling by having a smoke.

I've always felt that a person doesn't own the right to ruin someone else's day because their day isn't going as great as they'd like it to go, so I went with my roommate to have some Chinese food at a restaurant. We met another friend of mine named Jerry, and his wife, Pat, having lunch there too. I bragged to them that was my first day of not smoking, and Jerry told me that he knows I can stay not smoking because I'd already quit drinking and swearing and other things that were in my way to becoming a better human being.

For the next few weeks I drove people nuts by constantly moving around because I was as hyper as I was when I was a little kid again. It seemed I had to tell everyone I saw smoking about the dangers of smoking so I'd keep from smoking again. After a while people were offering to buy me a pack of smokes so I'd quit fidgeting around, but I kept doing the hard part of quitting smoking and never had one. I didn't know that fidgeting around was a characteristic that many TBI people share at that time. If I had known how great I'd feel after not smoking for a couple of weeks, I would have quit smoking years ago. After a few months of not smoking my lungs stopped singing (wheezing) whenever I took a deep breath.

I wanted a driver's license with no restrictions on it and sent a letter to the Motor Vehicle Branch to get one and they sent me a letter back saying that I'd have to have a doctor examine me and fill out the form they'd enclosed, and return it to them.

BC Medical wouldn't pay the $100.00 for this, and because I was so confident I could get a license without any restrictions on it, I paid to have the medical myself and had a doctor examine me at the brand-new Wilson Family Practice that had been built to replace Leigh Square after it was torn down. The receptionist told me they'd mail the forms to the Motor Vehicle Branch after I was examined. When the Motor Vehicle Branch got the forms and reviewed them, they sent me a letter asking me to surrender my license because my eyes and reactions weren't good enough to drive. I was so surprised by this that I relinquished my license without putting up any fight.

I was listening to the radio on May 21, 1987, when the announcer on it said that Rick Hansen (the Man in Motion) would be coming into Maple Ridge (as Haney was called by now) in a few minutes and he'd be in Terry Fox's hometown of Port Coquitlam that night. Rick would be spending that evening at the Best Western before heading for Vancouver the next day for the last leg of his journey around the world.

I was dozing asleep at that time and became wider-awake with the sudden realization that I didn't want to miss seeing another history-making event like the others I'd missed in life already when my roommate pulled into the driveway and walked in the house. I told him Rick Hansen was going to be at the Best Western in a few minutes and asked if he'd give me a ride there because I wanted to take Rick's picture. We got there a couple minutes after Rick had arrived and because I thought I had missed seeing him I started taking pictures of all the different Man in Motion vehicles.

The next morning I went to the motel to take a few more pictures before he left for Vancouver. As soon as I arrived at the motel I saw there were at least 200 other people with the same idea as me. I thought I wouldn't stand a chance of seeing him and started walking through the parking lot to leave. Then that inner voice of mine told me to turn around. So I did and Rick was right behind me working his way through the crowd in his wheelchair.

In late September, I rode my bike down to Hyde Creek Recreation Centre to watch the start of the Terry Fox Hometown Run because I planned on riding my bicycle around the route that everybody else would be running, rolling or wheeling. I must have been in the right place at the right time because I saw Rick at his car getting prepared to start the run.

That night I felt so inspired by what Terry Fox and Rick Hansen had done that I decided to do something about myself. So I went to Viscount and ran around the same field where I started playing sports on when I was ten years old. Doing that reinforced my feelings that I could do something about the way I was.

The next day I phoned Doug (the guy I'd met at PoCo in 1976 and had driven the van on Terry Fox's Marathon of Hope Run) and told him about my inspiration and got a few pointers on running from him because I remembered he and his older brother used to be long-distance runners.

Doug gave me lots of encouragement by giving me the revised edition of *Terry Fox: His Story* by Leslie Scrivener. When I read the book, I noted that Doug also gave Terry tips on how to run when he first thought of running across Canada. He wrote these words on the inside cover of the book:

"To Gerry,
A fit person any day now
due to Rick Hansen and Terry Fox's inspiration.
God bless you Gerry,
Doug, (Terry's friend)"

Every morning after that, the first thing I did when I got up was to walk a block from my place on McRae Crescent, over to Hastings Junior Secondary School (present-day Maple Creek Middle School) and run around the track there a few times. The book also told me that Terry Fox first started his running on that same track because he only lived a few blocks from it. I only got up to running a mile and a half before ending my running career because my left knee was bothering me a lot.

Chapter 23
Showing Up

Skip told me I should go and see his mom in the hospital because she wasn't going to be living that much longer due to cancer she had. I never saw her, and that's still one of the biggest regrets I have in my life today because she died on March 16, 1988, but her memory lives on. That taught me I shouldn't be so wrapped up in myself and turn my back on opportunities because sometimes tomorrow is too late.

At her funeral I remembered she always boiled her tea for a while when she was reheating it. This made me think that perhaps boiling tea after it has already been made wasn't a fallacy like I always thought it was.

Time moved me into being a voter at a Recovery function in Nanaimo, BC, in March 1988. While I was there, I saw a bunch of people in wheelchairs and others with different challenges. They told me they were from an acting company called Theatre Terrific in Vancouver and had done a few performances at that hotel. I told them I was interested in doing some acting with them and got more information and promised to look them up when I got back to the mainland.

I was hoping they'd say I couldn't join them because I wasn't disabled enough, but they didn't say anything because it should have been obvious to them that I was challenged too. In many cases one challenged person can pick out another challenged person quite easily. Being good to my word (a person is only as good as what their word is) I phoned them when I got home and I made arrangements to get involved with them as soon as possible. I did my first performance with them on the sidewalk in front of Vancouver General Hospital. There were only about ten or eleven people who saw it, but that was fine with me because I hadn't done much acting before (except for that scene I did as Ben Gunn in grade four, and the boxing match I did in high school) other than all the play-acting I've done in life.

That New Year's Eve, Theatre Terrific was invited to do a scene called 'Swami and Seeker' at the Third Annual World Healing Days presentation called 'Quest for Peace' at Canada Place. To add realism to the character I'd be playing, I went into the bathroom and doused my shirt with water to make it look like I'd been sweating for a long time. When I returned to the stage, Theatre Terrific's stage manager pinned a tiny microphone to my shirt. And when I started saying my lines they came out like this, "Oh Swami, I've been searching for you"… and when I moved my body all you heard after that was, "Shhhhhhhhhhh-hhhhhhh" whenever I said anything. Next you heard the other guy's lines coming out clearly. Then you'd hear "shhhhhhhhhhhhhhhh-hhhhhhhhhhhhhhhhhhhhhh" coming from me because the water I put on my shirt had shorted out the microphone I was wearing. It was the first chance I had to be on a stage, performing for what looked like hundreds and hundreds of people, and I blew the whole experience out an open window by trying to be more real than real.

I'd been trying to find Heather ever since I'd cleaned up my act and when I eventually found her we started conversing on the phone again. I ended up blistering the ends of my fingers when I started shining jewellery on a polishing machine for her. She gave me four or five vinyl record albums by Buffy Sainte Marie to add to my extensive record collection because I saw them in hers, and mentioned I liked Buffy's music.

A girl I'd graduated from high school with, and had done some piece work for Heather phoned me at my place in New Westminster, where I now lived, and told me about a co-operative housing complex in Port Moody that I might be interested in living in because the rent would be cheaper. To be eligible to move into this place I had to attend a members' meeting at the co-op in a couple of days. I went to that meeting, and Mom bought me the shares to move in, "as your inheritance," on December 15, 1988.

A different girl who worked for Heather now and again was excited one Friday in early April because she was going to an open audition for extras in an opera called *Aïda* at BC Place, 'a cattle-hall' as Heather called it. I hadn't even heard of the opera before, and never thought of it all day after I did. But the next morning when the auditions were going to be happening, that inner voice of mine woke me up earlier than usual and told me to go to that audition. So I took the Skytrain into Stadium Station and walked the two blocks to BC Place and got in line with all the other hopefuls. After a few hours about twenty-five of us were let in the building and we walked to the lowest part of BC Place where we stood on spots on the floor according to how tall we were.

For this occasion I made myself taller than I really am by standing with my spine as straight as I could for this important-looking lady who seemed to be picking people to stand in another group. I started staring at her and saying to her in silence: "pick me, pick me, pick me, pick me" over and over again to be noticed by her. Eventually she looked at me and motioned for me to stand in the other group. For the next few hours other hopefuls came in and were picked or let go. When she had all the extras she needed for the production she congratulated us for being chosen as extras for *Aïda* and told us where we were to go to get our security passes, our costumes and make-up done. I was now a Striped Man in the opera *Aïda*.

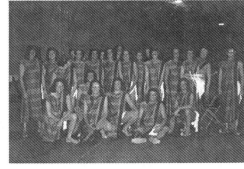

Aida's Striped People— first row last on right— sitting on the floor in 1989.

As soon as I was part of the cast I convinced myself the producers of the opera would discover I was brain damaged and they would kick me out of the play. But I kept this to myself and made sure I didn't do anything inappropriate.

My job at the three rehearsals and the two performances of *Aïda* (April 27 and 29, 1989) was to stand center-stage with all the other Striped People and wave at the Egyptian army as they were returning from war against the Ethiopians with their plundered booty of treasure, elephants, lions and tigers.

What a photo op that would have been! In fact, I brought my camera to all the rehearsals and took lots of pictures of people in their costumes backstage. I was seriously thinking of taking a picture of the audience from the stage during the production, but didn't. Those who bought the program from those performances took my name home with them because it was printed in it.

I was beginning to find that whenever my left knee was bent for any length of time it was seizing up on me quite a bit. So a doctor made arrangements for me to go into Eagle Ridge Hospital to have arthroscopic surgery in June 1989. While the surgeon was looking around inside my knee he discovered I had osteoarthritis, that I believe was caused by playing sports at a hundred and ten percent for all those years, coupled with the after-effects of my car accident. My left knee felt so good after having that operation that I decided to do things I'd never tried before.

One Saturday when I was riding in the back seat of Skip's car with his family after spending the day at a beach in Vancouver, the disc jockey on the radio said, "I'm down at the Plaza of Nations for the International Dragon Boat Festival, and the organizers need people to come down and volunteer an afternoon here." I gave what he said a quick going-over in my mind and decided I wanted to start volunteering again one of these days and continued looking out the car window. I noticed we were coming up to the Plaza of Nations that I remembered from my Expo days, and asked myself, "What's wrong with starting today?" I spontaneously asked Skip to let me out of the car at the next intersection because I wanted to volunteer for the Dragon Boat

Festival. This didn't freak him out because I've always done impromptu things since the first time we met. He simply pulled the car over to the side of the road and let me out of the car. I went over to the volunteer booth and told the people behind the desk what I heard on the radio and said I wanted to do some volunteering. Like any other TBI, a lot of brain-damaged people tend to think about themselves a lot.

While I was standing at the volunteer desk I thought that everyone at the Dragon Boat Festival would know I was brain damaged only if I said I was. Many TBI people tell other people about their brain damage in an attempt to explain away why they are like they are for a few years after their injuries, and the people they tell start treating them the way those people think a brain-damaged person is supposed to be treated like. I never said anything about it. They just took down my name and said I looked like a security-type person and gave me a fluorescent yellow hat and a white International Dragon Boat Festival T-shirt and was told I'd be stationed at a parking lot to tell people they couldn't park there.

There were going to be some fireworks when it became dark, so when one of the paid security people came in a truck to relieve me, he asked me if I'd ever been to the top of that huge structure called Science World before. Of course I said I hadn't. We went into Science World and walked up some stairs to where we couldn't go any higher, and after he opened a hatch I saw we were at the top of that golf-ball-looking structure. I said that would be a great spot to see the fireworks. He agreed but said he was afraid someone might see us from below and he'd lose his job. So we left the way we came in.

I liked volunteering so much that I started volunteering at every opportunity I encountered. I discovered that the people who volunteer their time are a different breed of people than other people because they want to get more involved in life by doing things for someone else for free. People who think they'll get something other than the satisfaction of doing something for someone else miss out on the internal reward one gets from doing a good turn.

A few months later when I was at the Vancouver Public Library when it was still at Robson and Burrard in downtown Vancouver, I came upon a whole section of sound-effect tapes that I thought an acting company might be able to use. I remembered once when I was on Main Street I had seen a sign advertising a play at Vancouver Little Theatre. So I went into that Heritage Building to see if they wanted me to make a tape of effects for them. There was a cast of people in the middle of rehearsal when I walked in, so I sat on the bleachers to wait for someone to ask me what I wanted. Suddenly the troupe walked out of the theatre for a coffee break, leaving me with a few stage crew people. It happened so fast that I didn't know what was happening but found out where they went and walked down Main Street to see if they could use a tape of sound effects for them.

As I was walking there their stage manager was walking back to the theatre and stopped and asked me if I wanted to have a walk-on part in the play they were working on, called *Screwtape*. It seems their director had seen me when I had walked in the theatre and wanted me to play a monk and act as stage crew during the play. That was another one of those once-in-a-lifetime experiences of being in the right place at the right time that I didn't want to say no to and didn't. I was only on stage a few times, but that didn't matter because most people have never even seen professionally acted theatre before. So I guess I can say I was a professional actor from November 21 to December 16, 1989, which proves to me that most of life is just showing up.

Chapter 24
Anything to Her

I've always had a hard time letting go of the past, and when *Screwtape* ended I had a hard time letting go of the fact I'd been in a professionally acted play and I started doing all kinds of stage craft things for the set designer. I did everything from painting the seats in the theatre to sweeping the stage floor before the performances for a complimentary ticket (a comp).

For Christmas 1990 Mom gave me a combination TV/VCR. A week later when I was at the new Save-On-Foods by Coquitlam Centre, I saw the Fiftieth Anniversary Edition of *The Wizard of Oz*, in its original format (in sepia tone—tan coloured) and I bought it because I had Mom's gift and hadn't tried the VCR part yet. I didn't know that movie had always been in colour because I'd always saw it on a black-and-white TV before.

A few days later when I was at a store I saw the two video set called *Woodstock*, and because I really enjoyed it when it first came out I bought it. When I played that video I realized the first and last performers of the entire concert were African American people Ritchie Havens and Jimi Hendrix.

That May, I checked out the Vancouver Folk Music Festival for the first time (that Anne first told me about in 1976). I met Anne at the first volunteer meeting I went to, and was surprised that she still remembered my name. A strong feeling of unworthiness made me think that she'd tell all the organizers of the festival that I had a TBI and they'd tell me not to come back again. They didn't say anything, so I went to all the meetings, and got my pass to get onto the site at Jericho Beach Park, where the festival has taken place since the second year. I found out it rained cats, dogs and sheep at Stanley Park the first year.

On the volunteer application form, it asked what I wanted to do at the festival this year. I said I wanted to be on a security team because I thought anyone could do that. What I didn't know at that time was that all security people do is stand in one spot for a long time or walk around the rest of the time. In either case, this would be too hard on my left knee, which was starting to really bother me a lot.

I did my three shifts over the 13th, 14th and 15th of July 1990 and decided not to volunteer at the Vancouver Folk Music Festival again unless I could sit at the main gate or something because it was too hard on my left knee.

After the Vancouver Folk Music Festival ended, I decided to look into taking a stage manager course at Douglas College, because the students at Douglas College are registered by their original student numbers and because the stage manager for *Screwtape* had impressed me so much doing what she did. I attended a six-session group of classes at the new Douglas College campus at the new New Westminster campus in it, and the class went so well that I figured it would be a cinch getting a job doing that type of work. But after I completed the course I asked most of the acting companies in the Vancouver area over the phone if they needed a stage manager without getting a bite.

Near the end of 1990 my friend Sylvia told me her son, Marcus, was going to audition for a role in *Jesus Christ Superstar*, to be staged at Terry Fox Secondary (formerly, PoCo) in May 1991. When I first heard what play they were going to be doing I was filled with lip fluttering and head scratching because the soundtrack had come out when I was still a student there.

I knew I'd have almost as good a chance as anyone else trying out for a role in that play because I had graduated from there, and because more than one person had told me to audition for the role of the High

Priest, Caiaphis, because I'd be perfect for it. I never auditioned for the role because my short-term memory was too short to remember to phone the school to find out when the auditions were being held. I missed out on one of those once-in-a-lifetime experiences I could have had but didn't, because my brain got between me, and reality.

Even though I was told they already had a stage manager and wouldn't need me I decided to stick with the play anyway and did whatever had to be done for the play because like I've already told you, I'm a sticking-to-it type of guy.

Another reason I wanted to give them a hand that year was because it was twenty years ago when I was the assistant director for *Hello Dolly* at PoCo, and if I helped the play out this year it would make me feel twenty years younger.

Looking back on it today, I see I forced my way into the production. No one in the cast wanted to say anything about it to me because I was older than them. The principal of the school at that time even remembered me from when he taught there in the sixties. Years before that he'd pinned an official Terry Fox pin on my suit jacket for talking to an assembly of grade-twelve students about what happened to me as a result of drinking and driving.

One day when I was sitting in the cafeteria, a 'jock' laughed in my face when I told him I'd once played wing in rugby for the team he was playing for then. Having him laugh in my face made me feel old for a little while, but I decided to toss that insult onto the bonfire of life by knowing that youth is still being wasted on the young.

After getting the list of cast members' phone numbers, the first thing I did was phone each one of them and remind them about the rehearsals every week. I stopped phoning the cast members in 1991 for the same reason I stopped calling the cast members in 1971— when I realized they were going to be at the rehearsals anyway because they'd already committed themselves to be in the play.

Some of the cast members knew I was trying too hard to help out or perhaps they were trying to hurt or teach me a lesson, because when a bunch of us were asked to move a piano from the gym into what used to be the music room when I was a student there, we had to lift it over a step and put it down on the other side of the doorway to get it into the room first. I took it upon myself to direct the way we were going to do it and I told the guys helping me that we were going to lift it over the step and put it down on the other side on the count of three.

After picking it up and moving it over the step I counted out loud, one, two and they dropped it before I could move my fingers out of the way or say three. After I'd heated a pin to a nice white hot and burnt through the fingernail on my right index finger, that finger released an inaudible sigh of relief.

In the last month of rehearsals it was decided I'd be a Roman Guard. I was only in three different scenes but it was enough to make me feel good about being in the play.

Skip and Bet came to see the play, and I remember Skip saying my name had the most stuff written about it on the program.

This is what was on the program:

Gerry Williamson: Roman Guard, chorus, Gerry graduated from PoCo twenty years ago clean shaven and forty pounds lighter. He won an award for helping out with Hello Dolly, *among others.*

A car accident in 1972 forced him to learn everything again. Seventeen years later Gerry was involved in Aïda *at BC Place Stadium, followed by a gig in* Screwtape. *He became inspired to become a stage manager and trained for one at Douglas College in September 1990. This is his first play since completion. He is still proving anything is possible if you try.*

The school even video-taped one of the performances.

A few weeks after the play finished its run I went to the school's Awards Day ceremonies, because I thought I'd win something for being the oldest person in the cast, but the only thing I won was the feeling of stupidity for going.

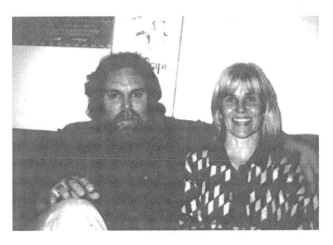

Full-bearded Gerry on my couch with a different Heather after the last performance of *Jesus Christ Superstar*.

When the Vancouver Folk Music Festival sent me a letter asking what committee I wanted to volunteer for in 1991, my left knee was feeling so good because it was the summer when my arthritis wasn't acting up on me, I took a chance and told them I'd like to work on the kitchen committee. I picked that committee because I wanted to get a glimpse of how the food was prepared.

On August 10, 1991, I took the ferry to Vancouver Island and hitchhiked to the Long Beach Reserve with a friend. We stayed at his grandmother's house on the reserve in Tofino—so we could go to a Recovery rally a few miles away in Ucluelet. I made a pest of myself to his aunt Nora, when I went into her smokehouse when she was in it, and stayed after she told me she didn't want me to be in there alone with her, which I'm very sorry for this today, Nora.)

I found out years later that many of the indigenous people just tolerated me being there.

It was quite an adventure hitchhiking after not thumbing in years. It was an even better adventure when Winston was taken into custody for an outstanding warrant for his arrest when we were driving around the town in his aunt's truck.

The RCMP took me to the rally and took Winston off to jail until everything got straightened out. My last day on the reserve, Winston dilly-dallied around by listening to the Doors' *L. A. Woman* CD over and over again, making me miss the salmon feast and most of the beach party that was scheduled there. I eventually got to the beach party and swam in the Pacific Ocean with everyone else. The ocean was absolutely crystal clear because we were the farthest west a person can go on Vancouver Island. I was freaked out that the ocean looked as clear as it did because I'd only seen polluted ocean water before. The water looked so inviting and the waves were so big, and it was so hot outside that I rushed into the surf without thinking about what I was doing. When someone who lives there told me that as soon as I started feeling dizzy I should get out of the water as soon as possible, I got out right then.

At Tofino in August 1991.

When I returned from the weekend, two of my friends, Sylvia and Redge, who had been worried about my welfare during the weekend, sighed a healthy sigh of relief that I'd made it back alive. Thinking back on it today, I was lucky to get back alive because there were at least three different times I should have been seriously hurt or even killed, but wasn't. Doing crazy things like driving a pickup truck along a narrow logging road to the top of a clear-cut mountain and roaring down the other side again, walking out on an old rotten log crossing a fast-flowing creek to take a picture, driving fast along narrow roads only wide enough for one car to pass through and not knowing if another car was going to be coming the other way or not.

There is a huge difference between having safe fun and having dangerous fun, and what I did that weekend was crazy, nuts and bonkers fun.

I'd already made arrangements to take a building service worker course for people with special needs at Vancouver Community College in September 1991. One day shortly after starting the class First Vancouver Theatrespace phoned and asked me if I wanted to volunteer at a bingo hall on Columbia Street in New Westminster— distributing the money to the winners, every Thursday night. The reason I was asked to do that was because I'd volunteered for them at the Vancouver Fringe Festival and had proven to them that I was a sticking-to-it type of guy. At first it was hard remembering who the winners were, but after I got used to it, it was easy. There was the odd time I didn't know who the winners were, but the winners always made sure I paid them!

One of the ladies who ran the bingo hall, Norma, was someone I'd met years ago and understood my condition. I think she explained my situation to the other women working at that hall because I had no problem with anyone there. But after she died and the bingo hall moved to a different location, the women running this new bingo hall weren't willing, or didn't want to spend the time it took to understand me.

I complained about this harassment to Theatrespace, but they couldn't do anything about it, so I quit. From that experience I learned that once someone thinks they have me figured out, it's hard to make their thinking face another way.

There were two 3-week practicums required for my building service worker class, that I did at Eagle Ridge Hospital. The first thing I did when I started my practicum was to move a bed to a different floor where I saw a guy I knew from New View. He was now skin and bones and couldn't talk from the ravages of cancer. I remember Dennis was a chubby chain smoker like I was at one time. Seeing him looking like that shook me up until I started working again because my mortality was shaken seeing someone I know being dissolved by cancer like that.

I saw my ex next-door neighbour from when I lived on Jensen Avenue a few minutes after I heard her name paged over the hospital's PA one day. Her nicker was Peachy, and I told her I'd heard her name paged. So she went to the information desk to find out why she'd been paged and I went back to making the floor look so shiny that people thought they were walking on ice and start walking funny.

I saw Peachy a few minutes later, and asked her why she'd been paged. She told me that her mother had just died and the hospital staff wanted to tell her about it. I turned off my floor machine (used to make the floor shiny) and gave her a hug. I'm not sure if it made her feel better, but I felt grateful knowing that Peachy wasn't working in a hospital where my mom had just died.

The last two weeks of my practicum started in early 1992 and went by without incident. After the last coffee break on my final day I was asked to get something out of a room in the basement. When I turned on the lights in that room a bunch of people from the cleaning staff were hiding in there with the lights turned off. They yelled "Surprise" when the room was illuminated, turning my mouth into a forest of teeth.

In early 1992 I started getting involved with a theatre company in the Tri-Cities (Port Moody, Coquitlam, and Port Coquitlam) to try acting with able-bodied people. I never seemed to fit in with these thespians but continued to stick with them anyway. In late September, that theatre company was invited to take part in a simulation of a major wilderness search-and-rescue incident to be staged in October called 'SAR/EX 92'—to test communications in a situation involving volunteers and other professional rescue organizations by the Vancouver Zone of the Provincial Emergency Program.

We were to meet at the new Coquitlam Town Centre Fire Hall on October 3, 1992, where we were given the roles we'd be playing. The role I was given told me my fictitious brother was in a plane crash. After we'd been given our roles we went away for a couple of hours to research our parts and were due back to the fire hall in character later. When I got back to the fire hall I created a bigger role for myself than what was called for, by walking around asking everyone I encountered what was going on and what I was supposed to be doing because I was pretending to be in semi-shock.

After a while it got boring sitting around the fire hall, so I went for a little walkabout around the fire hall and met someone I know who was a firefighter there. I fell out of character long enough to say hi to Chris and fell back into character because he looked busy.

There were big and small helicopters flying around with two victim assistance volunteers to assist the victims' next of kin get over their trauma. There were even two cameramen filming the events as they happened. I did some impromptu crying for joy when I was told my fictitious brother was found with only a broken arm and a few cuts and bruises. I may have over-acted because half an hour later I was told I wasn't needed there anymore and left.

Kwayhquitlam Middle School had already been built to replace Viscount Alexander and an open house was being held at Viscount before it was torn down. I arrived at the school early and decided to go for a little walkabout behind Viscount to relive and relieve some old memories. While walking behind the school, I saw an older woman walking towards me who was looking intently in my direction. As we got closer to one another she stopped walking and said my entire name as a question, "Gerry Williamson?"

It turned out to be my favourite of all time, grade-five teacher, Mrs. Horne. I hadn't seen her since leaving Viscount in 1966, I was freaked out she still remembered my name. I couldn't help but think I must have done something to her memory to make her remember me for that long. After we small talked for a while we went our separate ways into the school for our last look-see at it. I saw that beautiful dark-haired girl named Louise that I was so freaked out about when I first entered PoCo, and who has grown up to be a beautiful lady. Our eyes had a head-on collision, and it seemed she wanted me to give her some sort of sign I recognized her, but I was so freaked out about seeing her again that I didn't give her any sign I recognized her at all. I think she recognized me, but because I couldn't remember her name in time to say anything to her, I didn't say anything to her.

Chapter 25
Lunch Kit

A couple of months into 1994 a friend of mine named Gordon Watts asked me what I'd do with a computer if I had one. After thinking that I was born before computers became popular and knowing how much things have changed in operating them, I said, "I guess I'd have to learn how to work it."

"That sounds like a good answer to me," says Gordon. "I'll be at your place on Sunday afternoon to give you one."

On Sunday Gordon was at my door with a computer that had a colour monitor and a five-and-a-half-inch floppy drive. He gave me ten or twelve floppy discs and set everything up and showed me how to work it. Everything he told me was forgotten as soon as he told me because I was so dumbstruck to even own a computer.

If I'd had a closed mind when he first asked me if I wanted one I would have shut myself off from ever learning how to operate one. I wasn't sure if I still remembered how to get around on a keyboard anymore or not. But when I sat down to see if I could remember, I found my fingers dancing from letter to letter as I discovered that typing is the same as riding a bike—I still remembered where all the letters were from when I took typing in high school.

All I did for the next week was turn the computer on and off because I was afraid I'd break it. But I was assured it was impossible to break unless I dropped it or something. I did a few more things I'd never tried and the more I tried the more confident I became.

At first, when I wrote something and reread it, it was garbage. Like I was when I was in high school, my lack of self-confidence made me think of quitting writing altogether, but I realized I could edit what I'd written and fix it up. I wrote a few more things that were fairly good, and as time disappeared I was getting better and better at writing.

After two friends had dropped me off at the co-op after we had dinner together. Before they headed home to Mission, I asked them if they wanted to come in and see my computer. I showed it to them and Al asked, "Well, have you done anything on it yet?" So I dug out the floppy disc I'd saved something on and got it up on the screen for them to read. This is what they read:

> There was never a large voice that came booming out of the sky to proclaim life was going to be fair, but sometime during my teenage wasteland that thought did a dive-out into my subconscious thinking and has been clogging up my serenity ever since. On Awards Day in my graduating year out of high school I won three completely unexpected awards for doing things I thought were fun. I immediately slid into the idea that told me my life was going to go smoothly from then on. Then being armed to the nose with that powerful glory I tripped over a thought that told me my life was going to be protected by something omnipotent. I chose to dive into that daydream with all the ability of a high-diver doing a back flip and jack-knife can muster into one fluid motion. But the year after I graduated I decided to do some drinking and driving, but didn't decide to have a head-on collision with a bus the way I did.
>
> My life has never been the same. I went into a coma for fifty-two days, and during that month and a half I was out, I stopped remembering most of the important things I'd been taking for granted all my life. It wasn't as if I'd forgotten everything I'd ever learned as this tries to imply, it's more like sometimes things take longer to slip

from my short-term into my long-term memory than other times. Sometimes this happens quickly. Other times it doesn't. As it turned out, I have this brain damage that will never be going away like bad dreams go away. Even if a lot of the newer brain-damaged people insist on calling their brain damage one of those confusing contemporary-sounding names like head injury (which only makes the injury sound less severe than it is) I still call my injury brain damage because it's still damage done to the brain. Isn't it?

I got tired of confusing myself into thinking my brain was ever going to get better by calling it something it's not. After all is said and done, isn't a shoe still a shoe no matter what foot it's on? I've never been accused of being an Einstein genius before the accident, and luckily for me I'm not a quadriplegic like I could be today. Then again, I'm not like I was before the accident either. And as time drags its feet into the future, it doesn't look like I will ever again.

Just looking at a brain-damaged person, it's sometimes hard to tell there ever was anything wrong with them. It's sort of like a leg that's been broken; it spends time in a cast to heal, and when the cast has been removed, the person with the fractured leg limps around until the limp disappears. Then in about a year or so, you have a hard time telling whether there ever was anything wrong with that leg.

After the accident, I spent years and years relearning the things I'd once taken for granted before the accident. The simple things in life like crawling, walking and talking were all new to me. And like everyone else had to learn when they were babies, I had to start relearning the same things when I was twenty years old. And believe me it's harder on you when your body has grown. When I first started re-learning to walk again I found I had a different style of walking than I had before the accident. And after many, many years of physical therapy that style of walking is called a gait.

As a broken leg won't perform as well as an unbroken leg will, it stands to reason that an injured brain won't perform as well as an uninjured brain. And as a person with a disability you can't see, I feel I'm just as disabled as a person with a disability you can see. I find it strange that a person with a terrible gait will be hired for a job because they have that bad gait, while others who have worked hard to lose theirs, not only walk around without a gait, but without a job because they look too normal to be disabled in any way.

After working on myself full-time since 1972, it looks like the only pension I'll be getting in my sunset years will be my disability pension, and that ends when I'm sixty-five. I guess you could say I've always known my life wasn't going to be fair, but I never thought it was going to be this unfair.

Pat and Al both said what they'd just read was "really good" and added, "Newspapers would pay money for something like that. Why don't you send it to a newspaper and see what happens?" I was confused about this because I'd been thinking up stories like that for years and had never put anything on paper before. My family had never said they liked what I'd written on the notes I'd left on the kitchen table in my teenage years either. So I assumed my writing was lousy at that time and stopped writing altogether. Those comments Pat an Al made was the first time anyone had mentioned they liked what they read of mine; I wasn't sure if they were pulling my chain, rattling my cage or what they were doing.

So the next day I phoned a write-on friend of mine (a fellow-writer) because I trust her judgment a great deal, to find out what she thought of what I'd written. After I finished reading it to Margaret, she said, "At first I thought what I was going to hear wouldn't be any good, but you wrote something that was totally unexpected as far as I'm concerned. You've got your own style of writing, and I think what you wrote is publishable."

I asked if she had any suggestions of what I could do with it and she recommended Max Wyman of the Saturday Review portion of *The Vancouver Sun* newspaper and told me, "Send it away and forget about it." I fixed it up and the next day I went over to my friend Don's house, and he faxed a copy of the story to Max and I hid it away in my memory banks the way I was told to do. In about three weeks, or long enough for me to forget about what I'd sent away, there was a message on my answering machine from a Vancouver lady named Donna, when I came home one night. She said she wasn't sure if I was the Port Moody writer who wrote that article in the *Vancouver Sun* or not, but she could really identify with what I'd written. Imagine how surprised I was hearing that at 10:30 at night! I thought the newspaper would have contacted me before they published it, but they didn't. I phoned Jackie and Alfredo's place because I knew they took that paper. Mark answered the phone and he found the article and read it to me.

I thought my phone would start ringing like crazy the next day, but it didn't. Most likely because the people who think they know me didn't believe I'd written something that would be published in such a prestigious newspaper like *The Vancouver Sun*. Instead of letting negative thoughts wreck my moments of serenity today I simply turn them over to God and let Him worry about them for me. Doing that saves a lot of wear and tear on my brain.

A few months after that another friend phoned and told me that said she was working in the office at Lougheed Mall and the management there were looking for someone to do building service work for a few months. She remembered I'd earned a certificate in that and phoned me. Kimberly had already told the manager of the mall that she knew someone who does that kind of work and might not be working right now. The manager said I should come in for an interview at 3:00 if I wanted the job. I was there at 3:00 and got the job and started work in a couple of days.

While working at the mall, I got to know the security people fairly well and only remembered one guy's name. A few weeks after that, a guy named Scout and I went to see a couple of movies at Lougheed Mall. After seeing the first movie we went to the other theatre to see the other one. The previews were still flickering on the screen, so we did a bit of impromptu talking where Scout said to me, "Now, don't make a mess with all that popcorn like you did in the other theatre."

I noticed the couple sitting in front of us were listening to what was going on behind them and I knew their heads would be in our way when we were watching the movie and hoped they'd move—ensuring we wouldn't get a sore neck accommodating them. So I said in a loud enough voice where they'd hear me, "Yeah-yeah, I hope I don't get sick on the people in front of us like the last time either." The people in front of us got up and left after hearing that.

When the shows were over and we returned to his car, we discovered the car's battery had died. At that instant I noticed the one and only security guard I remembered the name of driving by, and he jump-started the car. Scout looked freaked out because it happened like it was supposed to go that way.

A few weeks after that Scout asked me if I wanted to scrape the old paint off a fishing boat and repaint it at a place in Richmond. The captain of the fishing boat told me what he wanted done and I scraped the old paint off for the entire day (wearing out the metal scraper in the process) and repainted it the next day using this special copper paint that stops barnacles from sticking to the bottom of the boat.

A couple of days after that Scout asked me if I wanted to go with him from Reed Point Marina (on the Barnet Highway in Port Moody) all the way to Richmond by boat, because the boat we'd be taking needed work on the engine. That sounded like an adventure to me, so I told him I was game for the trip. The next morning Scout picked me up at my place and we drove to Reed Point and the adventure started.

I'd never been through Burrard Inlet by boat before. It was another new experience for me seeing what the inlet looked like from the water to the highway, because I'd only seen what the inlet looked like from the highway to the water before. We stopped on what is called

Sturgeon Bank, where the Fraser River spills into the Pacific Ocean because the water was getting too shallow. What else could we do but sit and wait a few hours for the tide to come in and lift the boat higher in the water? While waiting for the tide, Scout jumps overboard to cool off. The water was only up to his chest, giving us a good indication of how long we'd have to wait. It felt weird sitting in a boat a long way from any land with shallow water all around us. We started getting hungry because we'd eaten all the food we'd bought at the marina, for the entire trip as soon as we left Reed Point. I said, "Hey, Scout, I can make out some golden arches way over there. You want a Big Mac?"

"Yeah, sure, Gerry," came the sarcastic answer.

Was he ever surprised when I handed him a cold one I'd bought the night before, from my lunch kit.

Chapter 26
The Day the Pearl Died

I've accepted the fact that my body must have taken more of a beating in the car accident than I thought it had. I also began thinking that the people who suffer from arthritis were not just saying they felt pain before the weather changes, because my joints turn into barometers before the weather changes today.

Mom started looking like she was having a hard time getting around when she walked anywhere. Using hindsight today, I think she had only been putting up with what she was feeling and not saying anything about it for years, because humans can get used to anything after a while. I found out that growing older is harder to do than I thought it would be. And I started believing that I'll have to continue being as tough on myself as ever because a person has to remain strong to get older. I understood that a person can only feel sorry for themselves for fifteen minutes and that was it. I was so far into coping with my own medical issues at that time that I wasn't thinking about Mom's concerns as much. She was going to see her doctor on almost a weekly basis and I thought he was taking good care of her.

Just before Christmas in 1995 I was walking out of a restaurant, and my ex rugby coach, Mr. Marsden, was driving by and stopped and flagged me over to his car and asked if I wanted to go to Lougheed Mall and have a coffee with him because he had to do some last-minute shopping there. After we got our coffee he told me that a few people from the Class of '71 were starting to make plans for a twenty-fifth high school reunion set for June 1996. At first I didn't think I'd been out of school that long because I believed that I was too young to have a twenty-fifth. But he proved I'd been out of school that long by using simple arithmetic. He even looked up the phone number of one of the people on the reunion committee and gave it to me. I phoned them the next day and was told they'd be starting to organize the reunion after the New Year and I was welcome to help out if I wanted to. I had a touch of scaredy-cats tromp through my thinking process because the other people organizing it with me would all be well established in their careers and I didn't even have a job.

Then I thought I was lucky even to be alive and doing as well as I was doing because I've met quite a few people who were hurt in accidents that weren't as dramatic as mine and are still stunned by the experience today because their injuries might have been worse than mine. That thinking reminded me that I had always blamed God for letting me get in the accident when I was still in the prime of life. When I digested that thought a little more, it hit me hard because I realized that God most likely grabbed a hold of me in a soft bear hug and didn't let go of me when I had that accident.

Using that power of reasoning today, and applying it to my new life, made me excited and proud to be a part of the reunion because I realized God had probably stopped me from dying when I had the accident. Then I figured that if I had the accident when I was forty-three, like I was when I thought that thought, chances are I wouldn't have pulled through it as well as I have.

I was so excited about getting the reunion going that I left my place in Port Moody for the first reunion committee meeting in Maple Ridge two and a half hours before it was supposed to start. At that meeting two of the people on the committee Siamese-twinned their minds together and asked me if I wanted to be the greeter for the reunion. I didn't want to say no to that request because I didn't want to make everyone think I had no confidence in myself.

When I got home that night I began writing the best story I could possibly write so I could impress everyone with how well I was doing compared to the way I was a few years ago.

I remembered that girl that I'd graduated with, who had worked a while for Heather and had told me about the co-op, and phoned her the next day to tell her about the reunion. Eileen in turn asked me if I was interested in posing as an angler in the fishing book she was writing. I told her I've been in a lot of people's bad books before, but that was the first time I'd ever been asked to be in anyone's fishing book.

I realized I still wasn't remembering a lot of the stuff that was happening in my life. I wasn't forgetting everything, I just wasn't remembering the important things in my life as clearly as I once did before getting the TBI, and decided to enter everything into my computer's memory because it would remember them better than me. That was the motivation for this book.

I accidentally let myself be manipulated into taking on a doctor in Vancouver as my family doctor, to have my left knee checked out before the reunion because I still didn't have a family doctor of my own at that time. This Vancouver doctor was the first doctor to prescribe an anti-inflammatory to me, which I was grateful for because it took away most of my pain. This doctor also referred me to an orthopaedic surgeon to have my left knee checked out. But, I couldn't see this specialist for another eight months and had to teach myself to grin and bear a very sore left knee until then. I started kicking myself in the rear as soon as I made this Vancouver doctor my family doctor because it was taking me about two hours to travel back and forth to his office by bus every time I had to see him and I was in such bad physical condition at that time that he wanted to see me on a weekly basis like Mom was seeing her doctor!

I noticed there were these little scaly bumps on my head, and red rashes on my elbows and knees, and was told it was called psoriasis. The medication the Vancouver doctor prescribed to me almost cleared it up. I remembered Dad had the same problem when he got into his forties as well. Everybody I talked to about this condition told me it was caused by nerves. I can relate to that because if there isn't anything in my life to worry about, I'm quick to create something to worry about. By the time the reunion was about to happen I was obviously favouring my left knee and when it arrived I was limping.

On June 29 (the first night of the reunion) I felt so nervous that the night would be a flop while being excited about seeing all those people that I hadn't seen in such a long time that I decided to walk from Coquitlam Centre to PoCo/Terry Fox to try and sweat some of the excitement off me. This turned out to be a big mistake because it caused me to favour my left knee the next night. There were already quite a few people at the school that I recognized, but there were lots more I didn't. A few people were intent on acting like they were twenty-five years younger and started pretending they were like they were then. I didn't act the way I was twenty-five years ago because I wanted to show everybody I'm a different person than that—I wanted to show everyone that I've changed in the last twenty-five years.

We went to the cafeteria where I did my speech and I ended it with: "I thank you for letting me be part of your lives because I thank you for being part of mine."

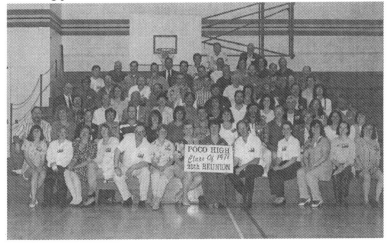

Class of '71 in '96—Second row left—photo by Preston Yip.

After that, we went on a tour of the school and we ended up in the gym to have Preston Yip take the class picture that wasn't taken in 1971.

The next night we had the dinner and dance at the Port Coquitlam Recreation Centre. No one showed any signs they wanted to dance, so I found Susan and the two of us had our first dance together. I eventually danced with Brenda to Janis Joplin (Pearl) singing 'Me and Bobby McGee' because I remembered walking her to her house in Birchland Manor the day the Pearl died.

Chapter 27
Like He Was

The food at the Vancouver Folk Music Festival tastes so good that everybody wants to keep eating it. So the kitchen committee decided I should go to the reserve table (a special section in the kitchen for the people who are getting off shift long enough to eat that meal and have to get back to doing whatever they were doing before that) and punch holes in everybody's nametags saying if they've eaten that meal or not.

After eight months ended I finally had my appointment with the orthopaedic surgeon, whose final diagnosis was that a knee replacement wouldn't be suitable for me at that time because I was so young. So my Vancouver doctor referred me to another doctor who prescribed a knee brace for me. A different friend of mine, also named Margaret, drove me to the place on Annacis Island to get the mould cast of my knee and then she drove me back there in another week to pick it up. The brace took away most of the pain but left me with an awkward-looking gait because the pain the brace left behind was too much to overlook.

On July 15, 1997, I got a letter from Asia Pacific Economic Conference 97, that asked me if I wanted to volunteer for them. The federal government was hosting the event, but the provincial government was staging it. I signed a form giving APEC permission to run a criminal check on me by the RCMP, which gave me some scaredy-cats because of the years of drinking, and the semi-blackouts I lived through. I mailed the forms back to them the day I got the letter and waited for a response.

Instead of letting myself get mentally messed up about volunteering at APEC or not, I volunteered at the Twentieth Vancouver Folk Music Festival on July 18, 19 and 20, 1997. On the Saturday I saw the beautiful as ever Buffy Sainte-Marie, who had written that great anti-war song 'Universal Soldier' in the '60s, as she was going through the line to get her vegetarian lunch. When I first saw her I remembered those vinyl record albums that Heather had given to me and wasn't playing anymore because I don't have a turn-table to play them on. I called Buffy over to me and told her I had those record albums and wanted to give them to her because the record covers were still in such good shape and she most likely doesn't have any of her own early records anymore. I told her I'd bring them the next day.

When I got home that night I spent a couple of hours looking through my record collection before admitting to myself that I no longer had them. I felt bad about that and the next day when Buffy and her manager came to get them from me, I had to tell them I couldn't find them. My big chance at making a star shine and I blew it!

On October 20, 1997, I finally got a reply from APEC 97 in the form of a letter that said in part:

"Due to an overwhelming response to search for volunteers for APEC 97, we regret to inform you your application was among those we were unable to place, but we thank you for both your time and talent."

I was ticked off at them for making me wait three months to hear that they didn't want to use me. It bugged me that they'd do something like that because I felt as qualified as anyone else to do any job they wanted done. I thought the real reason was they knew I had had a TBI and they didn't want to say anything about it to me. I wrote them the following letter that day because 'the squeaky wheel' is always noticed and given oil to quench its thirst.

On July 17, 1997, I received an invitation to join the APEC 97 team. I've been volunteering for different events since 1989, and since I was first asked to be a volunteer for you (by you) I've been excited over the prospect of volunteering. But on October 20, I got a letter that started out, 'Due to an overwhelming...' and ending with, 'with regret we wish to inform you...' I was devastated by this because I believe I'm as qualified to do anything any other person can do, except for looking Asian, being younger than I am, and not living in Vancouver, which are all beyond my control, the same as President Clinton's hair (who was the President at that time) being grey/white.

I'm still prepared to spend as much time as you'd like me to spend doing whatever you want me to do in order to earn a cap, shirt or badge that you'll most likely be giving to volunteers during APEC 97. I would appreciate a reply to this letter, thank you.

Bright and early the following Monday, I was phoned by a lady from APEC, and we determined I made a mistake when I filled out the form and sent it back to them. The mistake I made was that I said I could only volunteer for two hours a day when I meant to say there were only two hours a day I couldn't volunteer because I had to travel so far by bus.

I'd misunderstood something like that in 1996 when I'd written an article and sent it to *The TPN Magazine* (*The Perspectives Network Magazine*) in Cumming, Georgia, for their Winter, 1996, Vol. VI-I issue, after they had sent me a letter asking if I'd let them give my name and address to other brain-damaged people so they could write to me and ask questions. I wanted other TBI people to write to me so I could offer them hope that a brain-damaged person can get better.

From that I realized I should allow someone else who isn't brain damaged to read important letters like that to make sure I don't make that mistake again.

GERRY WILLIAMSON

This time, I explained what I meant to this lady, and she told me that two people couldn't do APEC anymore, and if I was still interested in volunteering for them I could take those places. I said I'd like that, and she told me about two information meetings I had to attend. At these meetings I was told what I'd be doing. After the training sessions were over I was now an APEC volunteer on the motorcade route. I was still sure they'd find out I was brain damaged and would tell me not to come back again! But I picked up my black blazer, APEC vest and green turtleneck shirt that the volunteers wore during their shifts a couple of days before APEC started.

I was still waiting for them to tell me not to come back again when we volunteers met at an elementary school near GF Strong for my first shift. I daydreamed about being shot and wounded, saving President Clinton's life and having millions of dollars put into my bank account by grateful US citizens, and becoming an international hero for a few seconds, before snapping myself into awareness of why I was there. As a matter of fact, President Clinton didn't even go by me that day, but that didn't stop me from daydreaming I saved his life though! I was stationed on a street corner on Burrard Street, across from St. Paul's Hospital, where everything was quiet and peaceful. Even the prostitute left her stroll because there were too many police there. The opening and closing of Burrard Street went on all day, and when the day ended a group of us walked down Burrard Street to wait for the army bus to take us back to the school. When I first joined the group that was congregated together, someone asked me how I felt my day had gone, and I said, "It was quite an adventure for someone from Port Moody to have."

There were about fifteen or twenty of us volunteers and Vancouver City police standing together on Burrard when I blurted out, "Sixteen years ago I would never have thought in a million years I'd be standing on a street corner waiting for a bus with a bunch of Vancouver cops." The police moved to the other side of the road to wait for their ride!

A couple of minutes later a few of us volunteers were picked up in an unmarked police car to be taken back to the school. I sat in the front seat and said what the Vancouver police did after I said what I said. There was a chuckle from the other people in the car.

Because I'd never ridden in the front seat of a police car before (I'd only experienced riding in the back seat—where there aren't any door handles because I was drunk in public) I asked what this keyboard thing sticking out of his dashboard was for, and was told it was a computer. From behind me came, "I guess that gives you guys something to play around with between trips to the doughnut shop, eh?"

The next day everyone was going to different places, but I was going to the same place because I was told I had done a good job where I was the day before, which also told me my responses to questions had been tested. In our training we'd been told to end conversations with 'civilians' (people who have nothing to do with the event that was happening at that time) when they started talking negatively about APEC, because the volunteers were the visible representation of APEC 97. Ten minutes later about ten or fifteen motorcycle police and an APEC 97 van drove by us immediately followed by another ten or fifteen Vancouver City motorcycle police; 'this must be someone important,' I thought to myself.

I knew I wasn't supposed to look at the motorcade when it went by me, but couldn't help but eyeball it for a few beats because I'd never been part of anything quite like this before. There were three APEC vans that went by followed by a couple police and other unmarked cars. Then a great big fancy tan limousine with tinted windows followed by a black van with an ambulance and a few more police cars after that. The whole experience was the same as watching any other limo drive by because you couldn't see anyone in the car anyway because of the tinted windows.

The last day of APEC I was taken to Burrard and Hastings where there were a lot of bicycle couriers riding around the streets. Part of my job was to tell them that they weren't allowed to ride their bikes on Burrard Street at all. Most of the couriers got off their bikes and pushed them along Burrard's sidewalks, but a few bad apples said the F word to me and kept riding along the sidewalk because I didn't appear to be a policeman to them. After a while my sensitivity stepped to the forefront of my awareness and I started feeling the lack of respect for what I was doing and began taking what they were saying personally. Then I decided that instead of getting myself all choked up and letting it ruin my day, I'd simply tell them to have a nice day, which would dish out a huge helping of confusion to them and clear any bad thoughts out of my mine.

We were eventually told there were no more motorcades and we weren't needed there anymore. So we thanked the RCMP and the Vancouver City police for letting us help them and they in turn thanked us for doing such a good job. We walked over to the Vancouver Convention Centre for a special thank you party that the federal government was putting on for us volunteers.

After having all the things we were carrying X-rayed and we had entered the reception room, the first thing I noticed was that there were tables and tables full of free wine and beer that I'd only day-dreamed about being allowed to have when I was still drinking. But seeing how I don't drink today I simply went looking for the non-alcoholic punch I heard would be there.

As we entered the room there was a short stage at the opposite end of the room with a table and chair on it. At this table was sitting this guy looking at the volunteers as they entered. Nobody was paying attention to him, nobody approached him or anything for the twenty minutes or so he was sitting there. Then Glen Clark (the Premier of BC at that time) walked from backstage and started talking on the microphone thanking us for doing such a great job of making BC look good and introduced the guy sitting at the table as Jean Chretien, the Prime Minister of Canada.

When the PM started talking at the microphone he thanked us for making Canada look good to the millions of people who heard and saw what happened during APEC 97 by saying, "As they say in British Columbia, merci beaucoup." He said a bunch of other things that made us feel proud to be Canadian and was gone.

I had a few more things to eat and walked to the Skytrain and went home. I met another APEC volunteer in New Westminster, who lived in Port Moody as well. He was all happy-faced because he'd shaken the PM's hand. It was nice to hear someone naturally high on life like he was.

Chapter 28
Not the Same Anymore

In late 1997 I had enough of going into Vancouver to see a doctor, so I put my choice of a new doctor into God's hands and took a doctor I felt directed to. When it was time to see a doctor I blindly made an appointment to see a drug and alcohol doctor in New Westminster because I thought I needed one of those kinds of doctors.

Mom had surprised both Jackie and me by selling the house on Jensen and moving to an apartment in the 1980s. Then she flabbergasted us by getting remarried and moving to a little house trailer. I thought that was one of the weirdest things she'd ever done, but I had to accept it because she was old enough to know what she was doing and seemed to be happy with her decision. I kept those thoughts prisoner in my own mind and never shared them with anyone by letting them become free-range thoughts.

Shirley always said she didn't feel very well after spending time at Mom's trailer. I'd take the bus over to visit her and found I felt the same way. On one of those visits, Mom told me that as she was getting older she stopped wanting to be with other people as much as she did when she was younger. In my own life I see I don't have to be with other people all the time either. But because I might say or do something that could help someone else in a way I'll never know about, I'll keep doing what I'm doing because sometimes it only takes one person or one idea to change someone else's life forever.

The knee brace that was prescribed for me had stopped being as effective as it once was after a few months because I was a big guy at that time, and the brace was made to support a much smaller person and was made out of plastic. This left my thinking sinking in quicksand that told me I should be used to the pain the brace was leaving behind by now.

One day when I was on the bus, I passed Lindsey Orthotics, and decided to be checked out by them and was told the brace I was wearing wasn't doing enough for me because of my weight, and was asked to get a referral from my doctor for a more supportive brace and bring it back to them. So I went to my doctor's appointment a few minutes later, got the referral and brought it back within fifteen minutes.

In another week when I was being fitted for this new brace, my effervescent (bubbly) personality came through and I was asked if I wanted to be the model when the Canadian Board for Certifications of Prosthetics and Orthortists performed their exams at GF Strong in May 1998.

Mom was like a lot of other people who had taken their good health for granted over the years and had stopped thinking she was getting older and one day discovered she was old. I didn't know that there was anything seriously wrong with Mom's legs until April 1998 when I was told she went into a hospital to have one of them amputated above the knee because she wasn't getting the proper blood circulation because she smoked too much for so long.

It appears that a lot of thoroughly dedicated or addicted smokers like what both Mom and Dad were eventually suffer from poor blood circulation as they get older. Once gangrene had moved into Mom's legs, amputation was the only cure to save her life.

I remember Dad's leg always falling asleep whenever he sat with it curled under his bum the way he liked to sit. He was always massaging the circulation back into it after a long sitting experience. I treated it like it was a joke at the time, but today I see it was no laughing matter.

Jackie and I went to see Mom in the hospital quite often after the operation, and one day when Jackie and I were in the elevator on our way out I started giggling because of how sensitive I am to situations like that. I was still in the throes of laughter when this large woman walked into the elevator. It probably looked like I was laughing at her, but the emotions in me were so strong that I couldn't control them any longer because crying and laughing are so close together that air has a hard time fitting between them.

I'd been waiting for a couple of years for a one-bedroom apartment to live in, and the day I found out that Mom's second leg was taken off I was asked to look at an apartment in the apartment building I wanted to live in. I was so messed up about Mom that I didn't even look at it.

One day I met my ex next-door neighbour, Peachy, who was now doing building service work in this hospital, the way I was doing it at Eagle Ridge when her mother passed on.

I noticed my right calf was starting to hurt me, and believed I had moved the wrong way or something and it would work itself out the way all those other aches and pains worked themselves out when I was still young and dumb and playing sports as hard as I was.

After Mom's second leg was amputated Jackie and I took turns visiting her with Mark, Steve and Paul (the boys) visiting her at other times. When I was taking the bus to see her by myself, I'd have to walk a long way from the nearest bus stop to get to the hospital. Doing all that walking aggravated my right calf and was making it swell up on me because my left leg was being supported by the brace.

When I'd get to the hospital I'd always get there when it was more convenient for me. And every time I got there that late I'd find Mom having her afternoon snooze because digestion is the hardest work a body can do. So I changed my mind about doing things for my convenience and started doing them for her comfort. I eventually timed my arrival at the hospital so she'd just get her lunch in the dining room, and after she'd eaten it, we'd go back to her room to talk. After she was put in her bed I'd rub some powder on her back because it made her feel good to be touched that way. Then I'd pull a chair up to her bed and we'd spend an hour talking about her past because her memory of it was still so sharp. We'd talk until she got too tired to stay awake any longer and I'd leave.

The phantom pains (feelings that make amputees feel they still have the limbs that have been removed) made Mom think her knees were hurting her. I first heard about these pains from amputees at GF Strong.

One day when it was sunny outside Mom was taken outside in a wheelchair that didn't have a wheelie or a roll bar on it. And because she didn't have those bars on the chair, she tipped over backwards and conked her head when she was going back into the hospital unattended. When I found out about this I was upset to say the least because any hospital worth anything would have made sure she had a roll bar on her chair. At least they wouldn't have left her alone to try and get in the hospital by herself. A bar was put on her chair after I raised a little Cain with the hospital staff.

From my own personal experience of being in a hospital I know that when a person is forced to be in isolation, their minds imagine all sorts of unexpected things are happening to them. Mom was no exception to this. She proved that isolation is the darkroom where we develop our negatives. The drugs she was taking for both her physical and mental pain from losing both her legs made her think all sorts of off-the-wall things were happening to her.

One day when I was visiting her she told me her legs were removed because she had cancer in them. My brain paused for a deep breath when she said that, and I immediately picked up a bag of worry that I might be a prime candidate for cancer as well. I was confused about this because I was under the impression that Jackie had already told me Mom's legs were removed because of circulatory problems. I mentioned what Mom said to me to one of the nurses at the nurses' station after my visit ended anyway. Mom's file was looked at and the nurse couldn't find any mention of cancer on it at all. The nurse and I talked about this long enough for me to put down the bag of worry I'd picked up and I stopped being so concerned about Mom's mortality and walked away feeling relieved, but concerned about her mental health.

Because I have one of those faces that show my emotions on it so much, the nurse I talked to must have mentioned I was all fuddle-duddled and confused about what Mom said to me to Mom, because the next morning Mom phoned me blubbering like a baby about how sorry she was for saying what she said and upsetting me so much. There she was in the hospital after having her legs removed, feeling absolutely distraught about how I was feeling when I was out of the hospital and feeling fine!

I felt I'd caused Mom a lot of mental anguish in the past, and now it was payback time for an outstanding debt I owed the woman who gave me my belly button that was a pleasure to repay. I felt I had to ease what Mom was feeling. It took me about ten minutes to calm her down and make her believe it was no big deal, and I wasn't upset with her about anything. I think Mom started to believe that I had my life more under control than she had previously thought at that time. At least, I thought I heard the shackles to my past fall off.

She'd seen me when I was sitting on top of the world before my accident, and then she saw me going through the years of physical and mental frustration of accepting I was in the accident. Then she saw me going through the years of physical recovery. And then she saw me going through the years of active alcoholism because of how sensitive I am. Now she was seeing I had a good grip on reality when it counted the most.

I think she started believing her life was a serious cross she had to carry around with her because she was being forced to look at it more than she'd ever looked at it before. The same way Terry was probably looking at his life and thinking it was never going to get any better in his last few months of life. The same way Dad might have given up on his life ever being different for him. She might have been crying about her own personal conclusion as well because around this time she told me she didn't want any big deals happening after she was gone. To me that meant she didn't want a big fancy funeral.

Something I've learned in life that's applicable to this scenario tells me that it's not the disease that gets you, it's the loss of hope that does.

Jackie and Alfredo and the boys and I went to see Mom at the hospital on Christmas Day in 1998. We had a nice visit and on the way out we met Peachy and I reintroduced her to Jackie. I recalled giving Peachy a hug when her mom passed on at Eagle Ridge and was glad she wasn't working in a hospital where my mom had just died.

On Tuesday December 29, 1998, Mom didn't wake up, close to twenty years and a month after Dad passed on, making me a complete orphan, and proving that a lot of seniors pass away between Christmas and the New Year.

Mark phoned me that morning and told me the news. I think there was quite a bit of concern about how I'd react to what happened because he asked me on more than one occasion during that day if I was okay. I'd halfway prepared myself for the inevitable, but didn't expect it so soon.

Mark picked me up and took me to the hospital where we met Jackie and her friend Ebba, who came to the hospital to lend her support. Jackie and I had a few minutes alone with Mom before we went for a coffee in the cafeteria while Mom was taken out of the room. After we had finished our coffee Jackie and Ebba left and Mark and I cleaned Mom's possessions out of the her room before Mark and I went and got some dress-up clothes for me to wear to the Mass. It was decided to have Mom's prayers said in the evening on December 30th and the Mass in the morning on December 31st to save the crunch-up of events happening on New Year's Day.

The morning of her Mass I got up at 8 am so I'd be ready when Jackie and Alfredo picked me up to go to the services. But around nine o'clock my brain took me under its broken wing, and when they came to pick me up I was still in my underwear. Alfredo did some terrific driving and got us to the church almost on time.

Skip and Bet, Sharon and Kay and Don and Carman came to support me. Ebba and her husband, Bill, and others were there to support Jackie and Alfredo and the boys. All the people I've talked to who were there have told me it was one of the best services they've attended. The Serenity Prayer was written on the memorial card, which some of my friends appreciated seeing.

Again, I didn't tell anyone when the events were going to be happening because I was too messed up emotionally. I later realized that what only feels like a few years ago there were five of us living in my family tree sharing the same last name, and now I'm the only one because Jackie has a new last name. It's like everything else in this new life of mine, it's not the same anymore.

Chapter 29
Just Been In

My right calf was continuing to swell up and cause me considerable pain. I started to believe that the swelling was happening like that because of the added burden put on it by my left knee being supported by the brace and my right leg being supported by nothing. Again I thought the swelling would stop by itself and didn't worry about it too much, but it stayed swollen and remained sore. I mentioned it to my doctor one Friday afternoon as an aside because the pain was starting to get too much to handle. He only suspected that I had a common problem that many people my age get called deep vein thrombosis and sent me to RCH to have a venogram to determine if I had one or not. A blood clot was detected by its appearance on an X-ray that Friday afternoon but nothing was reported to me at that time because the weekend had got in the way. And I had to wait till after the weekend for anything to be done.

On Monday morning, when I was still waiting for the results of the venogram to come back to my doctor (who would give me the results at my appointment on Tuesday because Monday was my doctor's regular day off) my right calf started hurting me so much I had to make an emergency appointment to see another doctor in the same office. When this more experienced doctor had one look at my calf he immediately said what the problem was and told me to go to the ER at RCH for treatment for a DVT. For the next two weeks I went to the ER at RCH to have blood samples taken and be given an injection of blood thinners to dissolve the clot slowly. Later that same day a doctor from the ER would phone me at home to clarify the proper dosage of blood thinners I had to take that evening.

I spent three or four Sundays going to different fishing bars along the Fraser River to have some additional pictures taken for the fishing book. I found out the hard way that I was working my leg too much, and my right calf was starting to swell again, so I stayed home for the next few weeks because I was told there was the strong possibility I could lose my leg if I kept doing what I was doing.

After three weeks of doing nothing the swelling went down but a pain started in my right calf that hurt a lot. I was prescribed some Tylenol three to take care of the pain. The prescription said I should only take six a day, but the pain in my right calf was leaving me with more pain than I wanted and I ended up taking the six T-3's and finding most of the pain was still there. As a result, I was always in pain and always tempted to take more T-3's than I was supposed to take because I have one of those personalities that stops me from being able to read a prescription properly and makes me think I need more pills than I really do.

One day I was lying in bed in severe pain, seriously thinking about getting up and taking a couple more T-3's when I started comparing the pain I was going through that instant with the pain I was going through when my osteoarthritis first started to kick in, in my mind. I realized both pains felt the same and I remembered I still had some anti-inflammatory in my medicine cabinet left over from my Vancouver doctor. So I got up and had some anti-inflammatory and within a half hour the pain in my calf was gone.

Because I don't like taking drugs, my doctor referred me to a specialist who prescribed a compression bandage for my right calf.

On May 27, 1999 I went to the closing ceremonies for PoCo/Terry Fox Secondary School because it had been decided that a newer Terry Fox school should be built and would open its doors to students when the school year started in 2000. The bus I was riding on went past the field where I used to play rugby and I noticed the crossbar on the northernmost goal post wasn't there anymore, indicating the field wasn't being used for sports anymore. I saw lots of people I remembered from when I was a student there. There were even two guys who remembered me from when I was in *Jesus Christ Superstar.*

I found out that the people who graduated in the 1970s were going to meet in what used to be the old music room when I was a student there, so I went there. As I walked into the room there was a lady standing just inside the door and I said to her, "I'm looking for the room the Class of '71 is in" because there was no sign posted on the door. She said, "It's probably in there" and pointed into the room.

My feet were hurting me because I was wearing a new pair of shoes I had bought that morning to wear that night, and didn't feel like walking to where she pointed to and started walking out of the room. As I was walking by the lady I noticed her looking at my nametag closely, and she said, "You don't remember me do you?" I told her I didn't know who she was. "I'm Rhea," she told me. I hadn't seen her since I went back to PoCo in 1976. We hugged each other and I asked what she'd been doing since I last saw her. She told me she had been a teacher at PoCo and was teaching somewhere else now. She asked me what I was doing with myself and I told her "I'm trying to become a writer." She said she was trying to become a writer too, and asked if I was writing anything now. I said I was writing what your eyes are reading right this second. We talked about writing as we made our way to the front of the room where the 1971 grad pictures were. All the comments I'd written for the annual were there below the pictures of the '71 grads. I was surprised by this and told Rhea that this was the very first writing I'd done that was ever mass-produced. The last thing she said to me was that she still had that book I'd given to her for her birthday. I walked around the school a bit more and eventually went to catch the bus; oblivious to the coincidence I'd just been in.

Chapter 30
Ever Had

On July 2, 1999, a friend named Phil phoned me to tell me he'd won two tickets for dinner on Saturday and breakfast on Sunday at a Recovery event called 'The Pacific Northwest Conference' in Richmond, BC. He wanted to know if I'd like to go with him because I probably knew a lot of the people there. I told him I'd go on the Saturday but Sunday was out because I wanted to go to a Japanese restaurant and have my birthday dinner with Jackie and Alfredo and the Boys. He said he had no problem with that and he picked me up at 9:00 am on July 3, and we headed to the event. On the way there I wondered if I'd ever been to a Pacific Northwest Conference with these Recovery people before.

I decided to look in this Big Book of mine that I've been saving name-tags and ticket-stubs in for years to see if I had ever been to one or not. I looked in my Big Book that night and discovered that seventeen years ago on July 2, 3 and 4, 1982, the first event I went to with these Recovery people was the Pacific Northwest Conference when it was being held in New Westminster.

That July 16, 17 and 18, I did my volunteer thing for the last Vancouver Folk Music Festival of the twentieth century. Being filled with artificial courage, I asked if I could pour the sherry onto the first layer of cake for the Festival Trifle, which was a consistent treat for the volunteers and performers for the last meal that the kitchen committee prepared each year. When I started pouring the sherry it turned on a craving to drink again that was stronger than I expected, and I had to ask someone else to finish what I started.

That same day I heard that John F. Kennedy Jr. died in a plane crash, 36 years after his dad was killed in '63.

The Vancouver Fireworks Society phoned me and said the Dragon Boat Festival volunteer coordinator had given them my name and phone number as a possible candidate to volunteer for them. They mentioned there was a meeting that night at a hotel if I was interested in volunteering for them. I went to that meeting and on July 31 I was stationed at a barricade that stopped civilians from entering Beach Avenue. My job was to make sure no vehicles parked beside a Milestones restaurant, near where the fireworks were going to be set off.

When I was walking down the middle of Beach Avenue a flare went up in the air to say the fireworks were going to start in five minutes and I noticed that the middle of the road was a good spot to watch the fireworks. Not more than a beat later, a lady asked me where the best place to stand to see the fireworks would be. I told her I thought that where we were standing at that time would probably be a good place to see them. So she and her family and I stood in the middle of Beach Avenue and watched the event.

At about 10:30, my right calf was starting to hurt me so much I returned my reflector vest to the other guy manning that position and started walking down the street to beat the rush of people that would be going for the bus too. I decided to walk down to Granville Street and catch a bus to Granville Skytrain Station. After I got to Granville Station I saw there were more than a hundred other people lined up on the sidewalk to even get into the Skytrain Station.

I was looking at all those people when I was suddenly attacked by a fit of impatience that I found impossible to resist and walked the few blocks to Hastings and Granville to get a bus to Port Moody.

When I got to the bus stop there was a cannibal's feast of people with the same idea as me there too. Four buses came and went that weren't any good for me, and I decided to walk the block and a half to the CP Rail train station that is called Waterfront Station today and take the Sky to New Westminster where I could get a bus to Port Moody. After I walked there, there were as many people there to even get into the station as there were at Granville and Hastings.

I was getting ready to throw myself into a fit-to-be-tied-up-in-a-straitjacket temper tantrum because everything seemed to be going against me. But I asked myself what would I be proving by doing something like that and turned it over to God to handle for me because anger is one letter short of danger in me. Besides, it seems that the people who fly into a blind rage always make poor landings.

I turned it over to God to handle for me, and that little voice that is inside of everyone told me to walk the perimeter of the crowd to find a place to step in the line and step in. So I started walking the periphery of the crowd and as soon as I did the sea of people parted like the Red Sea did for Moses, and I simply stepped in and went down the escalator and got into a Skytrain car and went home.

I was talking to a lady that I've known for years who knows all about my accident, and she told me, "You don't seem to be disabled in any way because of the way you've learned to compensate for what happened to you." That statement was meant as a compliment but that's not how I took it for some reason. I got defensive about my state of being disabled because I was upset that she wasn't finding me disabled enough. That was another change of thinking for me, because I remember when I was talking to the actors in Theatre Terrific in Nanaimo and was hoping they'd say I couldn't join them because I wasn't disabled enough.

That got me thinking that maybe I wasn't as challenged as I thought I was because I got internally defensive about my state of being a person with special needs because she wasn't finding me disabled enough. I realized I was holding onto my status of being a person with special needs like it was some kind of badge of honour because I have something that most people do not. I suddenly understood that I had figured out a long time ago that as long as I felt I was disabled that thought was keeping me challenged.

On November 14 there was a party at Jackie and Alfredo's house to mark their twenty-fifth wedding anniversary. To me it doesn't seem that long ago that they were first married. It was great feeling wanted instead of being tolerated for being drunk by those that attended.

My nephew, Mark, who is now a trained chef and prefers being called Marco today, prepared a meal that looked like a picture clipped out of the *Best Prepared Meals of the World* magazine (which is a magazine I just invented to make this sentence sound better.)

This was the first time that my Aunty Wava attended something that Jackie's sister-in-law, Barb, attended, so the three of us stood together because it's not every day that three people born on July 10th could be together at the same time.

At the beginning of December 1999 I was phoned again by the same apartment manager who phoned me to look at an apartment in his building when Mom's second leg was removed. After we had the interview together he said he'd phone me in a few days to tell me if I got it or not. A couple of days later he phoned me and told me that I didn't get the apartment because there was someone else in need of it more than me. When I was talking to him I told him that I'd move into one of his apartments halfway through the month if a vacancy ever came up. He said he'd keep that in mind. A few days later, he phoned me back and told me, that he had 'an early Christmas present for me' because the person who was going to take the apartment couldn't take it now. If I'd like the apartment he had showed me when I was at his building, I could move into it at the end of the month. Which would be the end of the year, the end of the decade and the start of the new century.

On December 27, Alfredo and Jackie, and Steve, and Paul came over to the co-op to help me move my stuff to my new place. After making two trips from the co-op to my new home all my stuff was moved in. I had packed a lot of my prized possessions into the plastic bags that groceries are put into and most people use as garbage bags. Because my brain made me forgot to tell the people helping me move not to throw these bags away a lot of my favourite stuff was tossed away because I didn't remember something important might be in them.

I went to a dance in Burnaby on New Year's Eve with a bunch of other Recovery people because the millennium only comes around once every thousand years. At midnight I decided to throw away all the keepsakes I've been accumulating over the years because those things were holding my thoughts prisoner in the past too much because I still have a hard time letting go of the past. I thought this would be as good a time as any to set a lot of my possessions free.

As time hit the start of the new century I began feeling the effects of what I had done in the sixties when I was still wild and crazy and what happened in the seventies when I had the car accident more than I ever expected. If I kept doing what I was doing before I had the accident I'd probably be feeling the way I was feeling then. But because I thought I'd done enough exercise in my life already, I decided to sit on my big fat past and do nothing and I'm feeling what I'm feeling today.

I've learned that when my arthritis starts showing me how much pain it can cause me from all those years of getting wet and cold in my boyhood, and playing sports so hard in my teenage years, and being in the car accident, and falling down drunk in my adulthood years I know I have to ask for help when I need it today because it's a sign of strength rather than a sign of weakness to ask for help.

I find that many of the people I meet in my life today think I have always been like I am today. I don't hold anything against them because it wouldn't do anything for me but keep me mad at them forever because like I've already told you, I have a hard time letting go of the past.

I began getting scared when my body started sounding like an old coffee maker inside my head, so I started seeing a rheumatology doctor. He prescribed some methotrexate medication in pill form to help relieve my OA pain in 2004. Surprisingly, this medication almost cleared up my psoriasis right away. I mentioned what this was doing to me and was told that it was a good side effect for me. I continued taking these pills until they stopped being as effective for me and was told I could start taking this medication by injection form instead, which I have done ever since.

In July 2005, the Vancouver Folk Music Festival decided to stop using the reserve table and what I had looked forward to doing all year ended. I was upset about this at first and internalized those feelings the same way I'd always internalized things I didn't like and never said anything about it to anyone, and started cleaning tables in the festival kitchen and quickly found that this was too hard on my left knee and knew I couldn't keep doing this for the entire weekend and let it fester away in me.

While that feeling was maturing inside of me I sat down at a table in the festival kitchen and started thumbing through the 2005 Folk Festival's program and got up to page 48 where the write-up on an entertainer named Utah Phillips was on and suddenly none other than Utah Phillips sat down at the table I was sitting at. This caused the feeling of synchronicity to flow into my understanding. I immediately told Utah what I had experienced.

Jackie invited me to a Thanksgiving dinner that was being held at Barb's house, so I was really looking forward to attending because I'm still overwhelmed about being invited to big family events instead of just being tolerated for being drunk all the time, by them. When we sat down at the dining room table, to eliminate any craving to start drinking again I've learned to simply move the wine glass away from where I am sitting. After a while Barb's daughter, Shanna, noticed there was no wine glass at my setting and like a good hostess she asked me if I would like a glass of wine with my meal and I calmly said, "No thank you." That might not have been a big deal to anyone else, but what only feels like a few years ago I would have said yes and drank my face off.

In October 2005, I took Marco out for lunch for his thirtieth birthday. After it he mentioned how fast the years have flown for him since he turned twenty. I couldn't help but recall what Dad had once told me about how fast time passes after a person turned twenty.

On February 12, 2006, Skip took me up in a Cessna airplane that he was piloting and we flew over Indian Arm. I was scared witless at first but instantly couldn't wait for the next time that I go flying with him. For the first time I saw what rugged land we live near on the west coast of BC. Now I can see how important that search-and-rescue operation that I took part in, in 1992 was.

I've realized that I'd rather regret the things I've done in the past than regret the things I haven't done because I've made friends with the knowledge that I had to fight hard to improve the quality of my life today. And I can appreciate what I can do today more than in all the lives I've lived before because it's not my problem other people don't accept me for being a little different than them because I'm still living the best life I ever had.

Epilogue

On February 20, 2006, my left knee had a resurfacing—where the cartilage surfaces were smoothed out. I kept my original ligaments, muscles and tendons. Again, the frustration of being a patient in another hospital flexed its resentful muscle in me by showing how much being a patient has changed since I was last a patient in a hospital. It also proved that the accumulated time of being a patient was as hard on me as it was being a visitor.

I learned that a lot of the other patients on the ward I was on were really sick and needed more attention from the nurses, where I was just sore. Thank you, Cathy the nurse, for telling me that.

Many people visited me every day, which surprised me because I still remember waiting by the elevator door in Lions Gate for people to come and visit me when the world was still revolving around me. Even M & M (Marco and his girl-friend, Michelle) and many others came to see how I was doing.

The physiotherapist at the hospital asked me to bend my knee as far as I could and I bent it till it started hurting and I stopped. I was told I'd have to bend it further than that before I'd be released from the hospital, so I put some of my rugby-playing will-power into bending the knee and bent it further than was needed.

Because I was one of the contact people for the Class of '71's thirty-fifth high school reunion one of the ladies in the class got in touch with me to give me the money to attend. I did something I was told not to do and the titanium rod fell out of place and my left knee would not straighten out and was taken to ERH to have it fixed.

In June my left knee wouldn't straighten itself out again because I again did something I was told not to do because of my short-term memory problems, and I had to go to Eagle Ridge by ambulance with its siren turned off. A very pleasant ER RN told me that her name was Esperanza and I somehow remembered her first and last names because they were such a unique combination of names. A few weeks later the same thing happened and I had to go to Eagle Ridge Hospital by ambulance with the siren turned off again. My ER RN, Kim, comforted my mind and my knee was straightened out.

A few weeks after that, the same thing happened again. This time I told the paramedics exactly what happened and I was taken to a room off the ER and the RN started doing what had to be done. She started hooking up an IV and I asked her what her name was so we could do some small talking. She told me that I probably wouldn't remember it anyway and said it was Esperanza. The memory of meeting her before jumped into my brain and I surprised her by saying her full name.

Then on November 4, 2006, my left knee would not straighten out at around 4:00 in the afternoon and I went to Eagle Ridge with the ambulance's siren turned off again. It was still pretty early in the afternoon when there was hardly anyone in the ER waiting to be treated. So the atmosphere was light. The paramedics were taking my vital statistics and I recognized a doctor who had set my knee in proper order before and he came directly over to me and immediately got my knee straightened out again. The paramedics were still filling in the report to pick me up at my residence when I asked them if they would take me back home again.

Somewhere in the space between being hit by a truck (in a crosswalk) and finding myself lying on a cold, wet road on February 16, 2007, I made up my mind not to be a grumpy old man and cause everyone around me to walk on pins and needles. I wanted to ease everyone's anxiety that suddenly appeared around me saying they'd be a witness for me.

I lay on the side of the road for a few minutes until the fire truck and ambulance arrived with their sirens screaming, followed by a police car pulling up the rear. I recognised one of the ambulance attendants from when he'd drove me to ERH when my knee wouldn't straighten out and had gotten V's name. I told him, "We have to quit meeting this way." There was no response to that levity. Off we drove to the ER at RCH.

The doctor in the ER had me stand on my left leg, both legs and then I almost passed out from the pain when I stood on my right leg because of the hair-line crack in my right pelvis.

I stayed in RCH until it was decided to send me to Queen's Park Care Centre on February 20 to wait for this hair-line crack to close up and the only way for it to close up was by not putting any weight on my right leg at all. The woman who manned the desk on the ward I was on had been the girl that called me in the waiting room of my doctor's office and escorted me to the room where I got my injections from my doctor each week and had suddenly disappeared. I had wondered what had happened to C. I stayed in QPCC until May 31, 2007, before I was discharged.

To be continued...

Printed in the United States
87725LV00002B/147/A